'This book is a much welcome contribution to the study of contemporary social pathologies. Based on analyses of late modern subjectivity, the authors present original and thought-provoking cultural readings of anxiety, depression and Alzheimer's disease. The book will challenge every reader to think anew about these phenomena.'

Svend Brinkmann, University of Aalborg, Denmark

'This fantastic collection of essays takes seriously Freud's observation that malaise in civilization affects malaise of the individuals. The authors show how neoliberal society today contributes to people's psychological and physical suffering. In a groundbreaking way, they link the rise of anxiety, depression and Alzheimer's disease to social changes that we are experiencing in today's capitalism. For anyone wanting to understand why people are suffering so much in the developed world, these essays are an essential read!'

Renata Salecl, Birkbeck, University of London, UK

Late Modern Subjectivity and its Discontents

This book analyses three of the most prevalent illnesses of late modernity: anxiety, depression and Alzheimer's disease, in terms of their relation to cultural pathologies of the social body. Usually these conditions are interpreted clinically in terms of individualized symptoms and responded to discretely, as though for the most part unrelated to each other. However, these diseases also have a social and cultural profile that transcends their particular symptomologies and etiologies. Anxiety, depression and Alzheimer's are diseases related to disorders of the collective *esprit de corps* of contemporary society.

Multidisciplinary in approach, the book addresses questions of how these conditions are manifest at both the individual and collective levels in relation to hegemonic biomedical and psychologistic understandings. Rejecting such reductive diagnoses, the authors argue that anxiety, depression and Alzheimer's disease, as well as other contemporary epidemics, are to be analysed in the light of individual and collective experiences of profound and radical changes in our civilization. A diagnosis of our times, *Late Modern Subjectivity and its Discontents* will appeal to a broad range of scholars with interests in health and illness, the sociology of medicine and contemporary life.

Kieran Keohane, Senior Lecturer in Sociology at the School of Sociology and Philosophy, University College Cork, Ireland.

Anders Petersen, Associate Professor of Sociology at Aalborg University, Denmark.

Bert van den Bergh, PhD candidate at the Faculty of Philosophy of Erasmus University Rotterdam, The Netherlands.

The Social Pathologies of Contemporary Civilization
Series editors:
Anders Petersen, Kieran Keohane and Bert van den Bergh

Breaking decisively with the often ideological and moralistic approach of treating problems of health and well-being as discrete and individual problems to be addressed in isolation both from one another and their broader social contexts, this series pursues the investigation of the ways in which contemporary malaises, diseases, illnesses and psychosomatic syndromes are related to cultural pathologies of the social body and disorders of the collective ésprit de corps of contemporary society.

It avoids reductive psychological and biomedical understandings of pathologies – including depression, stress-related illnesses, eating disorders, suicide and deliberate self-harm – to focus instead on the socio-cultural contexts in which they occur, examining the radical changes to social structures and institutions, and the deep crises in our civilization as a whole to which such conditions are connected.

The Social Pathologies of Contemporary Civilization thus welcomes manuscripts from a broad range of disciplinary perspectives across the humanities and social sciences – sociology, philosophy, psychology, anthropology, politics, economics and cultural studies, as well as from the fields of medicine social care, therapeutic practice and the healing arts – that explore the fruitfulness locating health and well-being not simply in the individual body or soul, but within a trans-disciplinary imagination that takes into account the integral human person's situatedness within collective social bodies, particular communities, entire societies, or even whole civilizations.

Late Modern Subjectivity and its Discontents

Anxiety, Depression and Alzheimer's Disease

Kieran Keohane, Anders Petersen and Bert van den Bergh

Routledge
Taylor & Francis Group
LONDON AND NEW YORK

First published 2017
by Routledge
2 Park Square, Milton Park, Abingdon, Oxon OX14 4RN

and by Routledge
711 Third Avenue, New York, NY 10017

Routledge is an imprint of the Taylor & Francis Group, an informa business

British Library Cataloguing in Publication Data
A catalogue record for this book is available from the British Library

Library of Congress Cataloging in Publication Data
Names: Keohane, Kieran, author. | Petersen, Anders, 1973- author. | Bergh, Bert van den, author.
Title: Late modern subjectivity and its discontents: anxiety, depression and Alzheimer's disease / Kieran Keohane, Anders Petersen and Bert van den Bergh.
Other titles: Social pathologies of contemporary civilization.
Description: Abingdon, Oxon; New York, NY : Routledge, 2017. | Series: Social pathologies of contemporary civilization | Includes bibliographical references and index.
Identifiers: LCCN 2016041016| ISBN 9781138213937 (hardback) | ISBN 9781315447209 (ebook)
Subjects: | MESH: Sociology, Medical | Health Knowledge, Attitudes, Practice | Depression | Anxiety | Alzheimer Disease
Classification: LCC RC455 | NLM WA 31 | DDC 362.19689–dc23
LC record available at https://lccn.loc.gov/2016041016

ISBN: 978-1-138-21393-7 (hbk)
ISBN: 978-1-315-44720-9 (ebk)

Typeset in Bembo
by Cenveo Publisher Services

Contents

Notes on contributors

Anders Petersen, Associate Professor of Sociology at Aalborg University, Denmark, is author/editor of six books and numerous articles. His main areas of research are: social theory; social pathologies of contemporary civilization; creative methods; sociological perspectives of the self; the sociology of diagnosis. His current research project can be followed at www.dc.aau.dk

Kieran Keohane, Senior Lecturer in Sociology at the School of Sociology and Philosophy, University College Cork, Ireland, is author/editor of six books and numerous journal articles. Research and teaching interests include social pathologies of contemporary civilization; the symbolic disorders and socio-psychopathologies associated with accelerated modernization, globalization and risk, including: ennui, anomie, melancholia, affective disorders, psychoses and the hysterical conditions of the twenty-first century; and as a consequence of this work, he is also interested in epidemiology, public health and social policy.

Bert van den Bergh, PhD candidate at the Faculty of Philosophy of Erasmus University Rotterdam, The Netherlands, with the support of Netherlands Organisation of Scientific Research. Since the late 1990s he has been teaching Cultural Philosophy at the Department of European Studies of The Hague University of Applied Sciences. His interest is in themes that are to be found on the interface of both philosophy and psychology – for instance, the theme of the contemporary 'depression epidemic' and the genealogy of emerging forms of subjectivity under the auspices of the 'neoliberal revolution'.

Dany-Robert Dufour is Professor of Philosophy and Education at University of Paris VIII. He teaches regularly in Brazil and Mexico, and is also frequently involved in various artistic activities. A key theme in his work is what he terms the 'liberal cultural revolution', a theme on which he has published several volumes. One of these is *The Art of Shrinking Heads: The New Servitude of the Liberated in the Era of Total Capitalism* (Polity 2008). His latest works are *Le Délire Occidental* (Les Liens Qui Libèrent 2014) and *Pléonexie* (Le Bord de L'Eau 2015).

1 Introduction to a series

Kieran Keohane, Anders Petersen and Bert van den Bergh

The series: The Social Pathologies of Contemporary Civilization

In *The Sociological Imagination*, C. Wright Mills famously claims: 'Neither the life [or, we would say, the health] of an individual nor the history of a society can be understood without understanding both' (1959: 3). In this spirit, the overarching theme of this book series is that the social sciences as well as the humanities should thoroughly investigate the ways in which contemporary malaises, diseases, illnesses and psychosomatic syndromes are related to cultural pathologies of the social body and disorders of the collective *esprit de corps* of contemporary society. Hence, focus should be directed at understanding contemporary problems of health and well-being in the light of radical changes of social structures and institutions, extending to deep crises in our civilization as a whole. Problems of health and well-being have hitherto been considered chiefly in isolation; both in isolation from one another and in isolation from broader contexts. This path has shown to have severe limitations. Instead, one should explore the fruitfulness of not just locating health and well-being at the level of the individual body, but within a trans-disciplinary imagination that takes into account the integral human person's situatedness within collective social bodies, particular communities, entire societies, or even whole civilizations, encompassing the health of humanity as a whole and our relationship with nature.

Social pathology was once a mainstream concern of the social sciences, but over the years it has become associated with conventional, 'old-fashioned', or normatively conservative standpoints. For instance, the social science focus on social pathologies of the early and mid-twentieth century was on specific topics, such as alcoholism, crime and delinquency and (what was seen at that time as) sexual deviance. More recently, professional clinicians and medical doctors have provided a great number of books in a 'self-help' genre oriented to both a specialist readership and to a broad audience. There is a wide variance of quality in the genre. Some are 'best-sellers' because their authors hold positions of authority and their readers are looking for authoritative guidance. However, the weakness of most books in this genre is that they concern themselves with one discrete problem – depression, or eating disorders, or stress – and/or that they are focused at the level of the individual subject.

Conscious of this problematic antecedence and its narrowly ideological and moralistic legacy, the Social Pathologies of Contemporary Civilization book series breaks decisively from this anachronistic context, as indicated by its three distinct emphases: the series focuses on the *social* – that is, historical and cultural as opposed to reductive psychological and biomedical – sources of *contemporary* epidemic pathologies; and, extending beyond the urgency of the new pathologies and beyond the immediate and particular context(s) of the present society(ies) in which they occur, the analysis extends to encompass principles and processes of global western *civilization* as a whole.

The social pathologies of contemporary civilization – depression, stress-related illnesses, eating disorders, suicide and deliberate self-harm, to name just a few – are the subject of much discussion today, and they are the problems recognized and targeted by mental health professionals and in public health campaigns promoting mindfulness and well-being. While sympathetic to these problems and while aware of these developments in public mental health promotion and appreciative of them insofar as they are well-intentioned, this book series is concerned with understanding more widespread social pathologies than fall within the conventional remit of mental health and well-being.

As well as these illnesses that are at least recognized as such, there are more general, diffuse social pathologies that have so far not even been formulated as being problematic. On the contrary, they have come to be seen, broadly, as the normal conditions of life in contemporary society, so much so that, echoing Sigmund Freud, 'to be sane in a sick society is to be sick relative to the society' (Freud 1961/1930: 102f). For instance, under the auspices of the neoliberal revolution whereby the norms of society are eclipsed by the principles of the market, a corresponding new type of subject has been emerging. Shaped by the experiences of hyper-individuation and the political-economic and cultural-ideological emphasis on the purported rationality of utility-maximizing individual self-interest we can see a florid symptomology of egoism, conceit, greed and narcissism that, in many ways, approach new forms of psychosis. Moreover, the amorality of the market and the relativization and dissolution of collective ethical frameworks and ideals (whether traditional-religious or modern-secular) under conditions of global post-modern culture, results in an amplified and intensified anomie and loss of meaningfulness, a moral vacuum experienced individually and collectively. One of the characteristic aspects of this social pathogenic milieu is a generalized experience of liminality; a morbid interregnum wherein we are 'stuck in a moment' as it were; living in a interminable present, with a lack of sense of history on the one hand and lack of a sense of a future – other than an extension of the present – on the other. Characteristic social pathologies of this condition of 'permanent liminality' (Szakolczai 2000: 220) include an acceleration and intensification of sensations (rather than meaningful experiences); a proliferation of choices (rather than significant decisions) and individual and collective amnesia/aphasia corresponding with loss of historicity, and of despair/hopelessness corresponding with loss of futurity.

Hence, social pathologies are treated as multiple and as being related to one another, and as not merely problems to be understood and addressed at the level of the individual sufferer but rather as to be understood in social and historical terms. Instead of addressing these conditions as though they were discrete pathologies, specific diseases suffered by private individuals as 'cases', the starting point is thus that the sources of these problems are social, cultural and historical: that they arise from collectively experienced conditions of social transformations and shifts in our civilization. This diagnostics of social pathologies of contemporary civilization suggests also a corresponding therapeutics. When we consider the challenges of recovery we realize that our individual and collective health and well-being will require more than changes at the level of the discourse of professional medicine, or at the level of the contents and forms of health services and policies, but, more fundamentally, a revitalization of our social, political, cultural and moral institutions.

This book series will solicit contributions of single-author manuscripts and thematic collections that address and explore different aspects of the Social Pathologies of Contemporary Civilization. As the theme transcends disciplinary boundaries, we call for several disciplinary perspectives – philosophy, sociology, social psychology, politics, anthropology and economics; from the humanities and arts more generally, and, of course, from medicine, therapies and the healing arts. The readership for the Social Pathologies of Contemporary Civilization series will be similarly trans-disciplinary and diverse, encompassing the particular academic readerships indicated above, and extending too to a readership in professional training for social work, nursing, public health, education, social policy and cognate vocational fields.

The series editors

Social Pathologies of Contemporary Civilization (SPCC) is an international collaborative project led by Anders Petersen (University of Aalborg, Denmark), Kieran Keohane (University College Cork, Ireland) and Bert van den Bergh (The Hague University of Applied Sciences, The Netherlands). The SPCC collaboration encompasses teaching, research and publications with partners in Denmark, Ireland, UK, Netherlands, Sweden, Italy, USA and Canada. The network has organized several international conferences and related workshops since 2010.

The first volume: *Late Modernity Subjectivity and its Discontents: Anxiety, Depression and Alzheimer's Disease*

This first volume of the series on the Social Pathologies of Contemporary Civilization, analyses three of the most prevalent illnesses of late modernity: anxiety, depression and Alzheimer's disease, in terms of their relation to cultural pathologies of the social body and mutations of subjectivity. Usually these conditions are interpreted clinically in terms of individualized symptoms and framed in demographic and epidemiological profiles. They are represented and responded to discretely, as though for the most part unrelated to each other; each having their own professional discourses of aetiology, diagnostics, therapeutics, as well as their taskforces developing health strategy and policy recommendations and interventions. However, these diseases also have a social and cultural profile, one that transcends the particularity of their symptomology and their discrete aetiologies. Anxiety, depression and Alzheimer's are diseases related to disorders of the collective *esprit de corps* of contemporary society.

Multidisciplinary in approach, the book addresses questions of how these conditions are manifest at the level of individual bodies and minds, as well as how the 'bodies politic' are related to the hegemony of reductive biomedical and psychologistic perspectives. Rejecting such a reductive diagnosis, the central research hypothesis uniting the book is that anxiety, depression and Alzheimer's disease, as well as other contemporary epidemics, are to be analysed in the light of individual and collective experiences of profound and radical changes in our civilization, of corresponding mutations of subjectivity and of the social hegemonization of the biomedical and psychiatric perspective.

First, before we focus on the three above-mentioned concrete malaises, the broader cultural context is explored by discussing the anthropological mutation of the subject which has taken place in the transition from modern to post-modern (or late modern) times. This mutation entails the emergence of an isolist precarious subject faced with the task of creating a self, though deprived of the conditions of possibility of successfully undertaking such a project under conditions of the neoliberal revolution. The presentation of the essential hypothesis of the mutation of subjectivity under conditions of neoliberalism by one of the world's foremost proponent of that diagnostic, Dany-Robert Dufour, sets the scene for the analyses that follow, namely those of three major 'epidemics' of our time: anxiety, depression and Alzheimer's disease. We choose these three conditions because not only are they key disorders of our present age, but also they correspond roughly with stages of the life course, anxiety being the fastest-growing malaise among youth and adolescence; depression being an affliction especially of young adulthood and mid-life; and Alzheimer's dementia as the coming 'epidemic' of an aging population.

So first, in Chapter 2, the French philosopher Dany-Robert Dufour outlines the context of late modern social pathologies by focusing on the transition from modern to post-modern (or late modern) subjectivity. In the last 15 years Dufour has undertaken an extensive, multi-volume investigation into what he terms the 'liberal cultural revolution', a cultural transformation the heart of which consists in a gradual, longlasting liberation of the human passions, leading to the emergence of a Sadean, isolist type of subject. 'Isolism' is a term De Sade used to indicate his ideal type of individual: narcissist and hedonist. According to Dufour, it is this type of subject which is propagated, stimulated and constituted by late modern capitalism, or, in other words, by the 'Divine

Market'. Here, in this second chapter of this first volume of our series, Dufour's analysis of the 'anthropological mutation' proceeds in in four steps. First, he reveals his psychoanalytical sources by defining the subject-as-such as the being that because of its neotenic nature is the 'most-low' (or the little subject) who is subject to the 'Most-High' (or the big Subject, or the Other). Second, while working within the Lacanian psychoanalytic paradigm Dufour critiques and develops that paradigm by presenting what the latter fails to take properly into account, namely the different historical, anthropological, sociological and political figures of the big Subject: these include totems, spirits, immanent gods, transcendent gods; sundry kings and absolute monarchs; and, more recently, modern iterations and incarnations of the big Other such as the nation, the people, the great leader; or abstractions such as reason and science; and, finally, today, the market, which – in Dufour's account – purports to be a big Subject, but it fails to be such. Third, Dufour separates modernity, which he presents as the space in which the subject is defined by several figures of the big Subject, from post-modernity, in which the grand narratives have collapsed and no other presentable figures of the big Subject can be proposed. The market is inadequate as a new big Subject, Dufour states, because it doesn't function as a 'grand story' – that is, not as an encompassing collective narrative – but as a fragmented whole of ego-oriented 'small stories'. Therefore it has nothing to offer to the subject considering the basic problem of foundation. It only offers dual relationships and does not acknowledge the third. In this way it confronts the subject with the impossible task of founding itself. The subject henceforth is defined auto-referentially instead of hetero-referentially. The result of this is a mutation of subjectivity: the modern neurotic and critical subject makes way for the post-modern 'psychotisizing' or borderline-like subject, which is no longer functioning primarily symbolically but libidinally. This dynamized insecure auto-referential subject is an easy target for the powerful apparatus called the market. 'Neoliberal' times are therefore the era of a new servitude. Lastly, Dufour discusses briefly ways of compensating for the absence of the big Subject: 1) groups and gangs, 2) sects, 3) dependence and addiction, 4) omnip otence and 5) depression.

After this, in Chapter 3, Anders Petersen presents the thesis of a return of the 'age of anxiety'. Since the end of the 1980s we have lived in what Jerome Wakefield and Allan V. Horwitz have referred to as the 'age of depression'. Their claim is based on two facts: first, that during the last 30–40 years, more and more people have been diagnosed with depression; second, that western countries particularly have witnessed a steep increase in the number of people who use antidepressant medication. Although depression is still a very common diagnosis – and medicalization of mental illnesses such as depression has not come to an end – there seems to have been a development towards anxiety as becoming the more precise signifier of our contemporary mental malaise. Empirically, this is backed by recent statistics that show that anxiety has dethroned depression as the most commonly diagnosed mental disorder in Denmark (and elsewhere). Now, W.H. Auden famously proclaimed in the

1950s that this was 'the age of anxiety' – so one should perhaps talk about the return of that particular age. But, one cannot equate Auden's age of anxiety with the one that seems to haunt contemporary life. The general claim in this chapter is that there are different types of anxiety at stake today than in Auden's age and that anxiety should be seen as a particular social pathology that reveals particular aspects of contemporary society.

In Chapter 4 Bert van den Bergh discusses a phenomenon that only since 1980 has been formally separated from anxiety, namely depression. On the basis of, among other things, Dufour's analysis of the 'liberal cultural revolution' and his identification of a 'Sadean subject', the focus in this chapter is on the so-called 'depression epidemic', which is said to be haunting late modernity. According to the World Health Organization (WHO), depression is 'the leading cause of disability world-wide'. Within the dominant *Diagnostic and Statistical Manual of Mental Disorders* (*DSM*)-based conceptual and practical framework of mental health care this disorder is taken as a universal condition which particularly hits our contemporary society. In this chapter this presupposition is questioned by taking a cross-cultural perspective. The leading thesis is as follows: the phenomenon which we have termed 'depression' is not only *interpreted* but also *constituted* differently across cultures because of the 'work of culture' – that is, culture-specific narratives and practices. This thesis is explored via a discussion of the critique that has been formulated from different theoretical angles on the concept of depression as it dominates western mental health care discourses since the 'neo-Kraepelinian revolution' of *DSM-III* in 1980. The chapter moves from a critique from the (biopsychiatric) 'inside' to one from the (phenomenological) 'outside'. Taking the dominant *DSM*-based interpretation of depression as a culture-specific and historically determined understanding of a universal underlying phenomenon leads to the twofold question of what this underlying phenomenon might be and how we may get access to it. A preliminary answer to these questions is that we need to 'bracket' our dominant understanding of 'depression' in order to get to the *Sache selbst* – that is to say, this 'mental disorder' understood on the level of (a disruption of) a primal process of preconscious attunement by a presubject and its ambiance. Bracketing our dominant understanding of depression means turning away from the 'neoliberal', (hyper)individualistic interpretation of subjectivity and getting back to the human being as basically a 'social animal'. From a phenomenological, non-individualistic angle depression then comes to the fore as a *social* affect and as a disruption of a basic *attunement*. The depressed individual, in other words, is above all not sad but *isolated* or *distuned*.

The third concrete malaise that is discussed by Kieran Keohane in Chapter 5 is Alzheimer's disease. The general hypothesis is that what has come to be known as 'Alzheimer's disease' arises from the unfulfilled deep need for life to be coherent and meaningful. Alzheimer's disease and the dementia reputed to it are formulated in terms of transformations of late modern society, the disintegration of individual consciousness from the *conscience collective* and fragmentation of the symbolic order resulting in generalized *asymbolia* (loss of meaningfulness).

The analysis is developed by re-examining the findings of the 'Nun Study', the most famous longitudinal epidemiology of Alzheimer's disease to date. These empirical materials are reformulated in terms of classical and contemporary social theory, notably Durkheim, on individuation and transformation of the *conscience collective* as defining experiences of modernization, and Weber, on the centrality of *Beruf* – fulfilling a life task in pursuit of a 'vocation', which is echoed in Antonovsky's identification of the importance of 'sense of coherence' to 'salutogenesis'. These themes are elaborated through contemporary perspectives derived from Dany-Robert Dufour (on the symbolic orders of post-modernism and neoliberalism); Charles Taylor (on changing 'sources of the self'); Hartmut Rosa (on the experience of social acceleration), among others, to argue that Alzheimer's disease and the dementia reputed to it should be understood as a social pathology of contemporary civilization arising from the loss of stable bases from which coherent, meaningful life projects can be conducted.

In Chapter 6, finally, the three authors of this volume will look into a possible future of the SPCC project. Having presented one of the foundational theoretical formulations of the sources of the malaise of our age by Dany-Robert Dufour, followed by three particular studies of the characteristic social pathologies associated with the symbolic and anthropological mutations of the age of the neoliberal revolution – anxiety, depression and Alzheimer's disease – we return in this section to broaden the horizon again to a more general perspective, intended to set a research agenda for the whole project, namely studies in the social pathologies of contemporary civilization. That entails identifying and providing initial formulations, working hypotheses and fruitful metaphors regarding some of the characteristic current malaises, discontents and sources of distress experienced in everyday life by late modern subjects, including, but not limited to: new modalities of alienation and reification in the work–life experience; diffuse experiences of loss of meaningfulness; worries about selfhood and representations of the self in the contexts of the boundless social mediascapes; manifestations of pleonexic excess of appetites and desires, distunements and dysrhythmias in libidinal and political economies due to loss of anthropological ground and transcendent limits. As well as flagging some of the forthcoming themes in the book series, we will also focus on prophylactics, healthy responses and hopeful and creative adaptations to the malaises of our age.

References

Freud, S. (1961/1930): *Civilization and its Discontents*. New York: Norton.
Szakolczai, A. (2000): *Reflexive Historical Sociology*. London: Routledge.
Wright Mills, C. (1959): *The Sociological Imagination*. Oxford: Oxford University Press.

2 Modern subjectivity/ post-modern subjectivity

Dany-Robert Dufour

In this chapter I would like to discuss post-modern subjectivity, and how it differs from modern subjectivity. I shall first describe what I understand by subjectivity, then I shall attempt to show that this subjectivity varies historically and also explore a hypothesis which I have already worked on extensively, namely that there has been a recent, major and decisive change in this subjectivity. Lastly, I will relate consequences of this mutation to certain recent 'socio-pathological' incidents.

The subject, in sub-mission

What do I understand by 'subjectivity'? The concept refers, of course, to the term 'subject', which today designates a person who is a bearer of rights and obligations, as in the expression 'legal subject'. But we should not forget that behind this recent definition lurks an older one, derived from the Latin *subjectus*, which designates the state of someone who is *subjected*, in *sub-mission* [*soumis*]. So let us start from this definition, that the subject is first and foremost subjected. This immediately raises two questions. First, why is the subject subjected? And second, to what is the subject subjected?

Why is the subject subjected? Because it is incomplete and imperfect. And this for two reasons. The first reason can be called *ontological*: the subject is subjected to finitude in time and in space: we are all finite beings in space (each of us is under a kind of 'house arrest', I mean confined to a particular space, here and not there); and we are all finite in time (for each of us, an end will come – I hope I am not bringing you terribly bad news). The subject is incomplete and imperfect for a second reason, which we can call *ontic* or *anthropological*: we are not only subjected to finitude in time and in space, we additionally enter this world unfinished. The human being is the only higher mammal to be born so notoriously incomplete. This species-typical prematurity, as it is called, is visible in a range of deficiencies at birth: the heart's *ductus arteriosus* is not closed, neural pathways through the pyramidal tract are underdeveloped, the lung's alveolae are inadequate, the skull plates are not closed up (fontanelles), the brain folds are poorly developed, the opposable back thumb is absent, as are body hair and milk teeth, not to mention, in the male of the species, the absence of the penis bone or *os penis* – which is sometimes very regrettable. Human beings are born premature, and they require a very long period of care. Although they are capable of reproducing and transmitting the juvenile characteristics which, with other animals, are only temporary, they are incapable of attaining full seminal development.

Our awareness of the human being's essential prematurity is nothing new. In an earlier work, I endeavoured to show that a whole field of study devoted to the issue of the originary incompleteness of the human being has existed since the dawn of western civilization (Dufour 1999, cf 2005, 2012). Western metaphysics, whether stemming from Athens or Jerusalem, has identified the human being's affliction, at birth and in early childhood, as the decisive source of the human being's journey. And this field of study happens to be rooted in the real, insofar as, since the beginning of the twentieth century, anthropologists have been talking of humankind's 'neoteny', its essential prematurity.

So that is where the adventure of the human subject begins, with an incompletely formed being who is incapable of pulling through alone, and whom I will call the most-low [*le très-bas*]. The German term used by Sigmund Freud to designate this originary affliction is *Hilflosigkeit*. It is remarkable that this concept should glint out at us across the whole of Freud's work. For example, the human being's prematurity is explicitly referred to in the 1926 text *Inhibitions, Symptoms and Anxiety*:

> Among the factors that play a part in the causation of neuroses … is the long period of time during which the young of the human species is in a condition of helplessness [*Hilflosigkeit* in German] and dependence. Its intra-uterine existence seems to be short in comparison with that of most animals, and it is sent into the world in a less finished state.
>
> Freud 1948/1926: 186

This prematurity is central to Freud's thinking, and it generates a whole new construction of the neuroses. Of the three essential factors Freud cites to explain how the neuroses come about, the most important one is the biological factor – that is, the infant's state of helplessness and dependence, which is unambiguously linked to his prematurity at birth. Freud states: 'The biological factor, then, establishes the earliest situations of danger and creates the need to be loved which will accompany the child through the rest of its life' (ibid.: 186f). Freud's argument is, in essence, that this prematurity creates the need for love which in turn gives rise to neurosis.

Where did Freud get this term from? Now, I have a guilty pleasure to share with you: my fondness for theological research. In this pursuit, I discovered, one day, that the term *Hilflosigkeit* comes from German theological texts, specifically Luther, who makes abundant use of the term *Hilfe*, meaning 'help', the help of God in this case, and how necessary it is for the salvation of man, that *hilf-los* one (that is, the one *deprived* of *Hilfe*), the one who is so low. So low, indeed, that in a famous sermon Luther went so far as to compare humankind to 'waste matter which falls into the world from the devil's anus' (Lacan 1992: 93) – which presents us with the very exact opposite of man as king of God's creation. Neoteny, *Hilflosigkeit*, thus generates a need for love which can extend to need for the love of God.

This leads me to the second question I asked at the outset: to what is the subject, the most-low, subjected? Reply: to the Most-High. I, who am a finite being in time and in space, who enter the world so incomplete, I can find some kind of antidote to this if I posit the existence of an infinite being, to whom I owe everything. And I am quite capable of imagining this being because my capacity to speak is also a capacity to invent fables, and hence nothing prevents me from inventing in speech something which has no existence at all in the real but which is a life-line for me. For if I suppose that he, the Most-High, the supreme Subject, exists, then I can *sub-ject* myself to him as his subject. And this is precisely what is meant by 'subject', as I stated at the outset: being 'sub-jected', thrown under. It is necessary – and sufficient – for me to dream up a *big Subject, supposed to be all-knowing, all-powerful and all-seeing*; I will be able at last to find my place as subject of this being. This big Subject corresponds to Aristotle's definition in the *Metaphysics* of 'the one on whom all else depends'. In other words, human beings are a strange sort of unfinished animal, who, unlike other animals, must bring themselves to completion, not in their *first nature*, but in their *second nature*, generally called *culture*. At the heart of this culture is enthroned the Subject, capital 'S'.

In other words, the survival of this prematurely born animal, the human being, who is deficient by nature, is predicated on the creation of super-natural beings: I mean beings of culture who, although inexistent, feature a powerful symbolic efficiency. But creating super-natural beings is terribly tiring. One has to mobilize all the resources of auditory, visual and narrative representation in order to endow this absent big Subject with a style, a form, a voice, a history and a place of abode because it must be represented, including as an un-representable. In other words, it is art (narratives, music and visual arts) which creates the big Subject. Or even: art is the art of creating the big Subject. What is lacking in nature is invented in culture through language, texts, artistic works, through myths and so forth. Aristotle had already sensed this when he wrote that 'art partly completes what nature cannot bring to a finish, and partly imitates her' (Aristotle 1966: *Physica* II–VIII 199a 15–17). We can speak here of the work of culture: it brings simply subjectivation. Once this big Subject is erected, the fundamental structure of subjectivation is in place, with the little subject below and the big Subject above. One can say, therefore, that the assumption of subjectivity is predicated on the supposition of a big Subject, which must precisely be written with a capital 'S'.

This symbolic remedy for humankind's real affliction partakes of what Plato calls a *pharmakon*: *both* a cure *and* a poison. That is why, this big Subject who does not exist, is extremely helpful, until it becomes … extremely burdensome. The supposition of the big Subject is a *cure* because it rescues me from my originary destitution, but it is also a *poison* because it alienates me in the big

Subject. As Freud maintained, this structure produces neurosis, or, to put it differently, neurosis results from one's symbolic debt to the big Subject. This leads me to certain clinical considerations.

Neurosis is generated by this structure because it leads me to believe that, in this world in which I find myself, I owe everything to the big Subject, who has given me everything. And two gifts in particular: one real gift, that of life, and the other a symbolic gift, that of language. Both are so exorbitantly precious that I will never be able to pay back my debt. And I will therefore always feel guilty.

Hysteria is the prototype of neurosis because hysterics both adore the big Subject who has given them everything and, at the same time, detest this big Subject for having created the situation in which they owe absolutely everything to it. They love the big Subject while hating it, or hate the big Subject while loving it. This constitutes a major psychical node in which neurotic conflict is constantly revived in all its forms. The hysteric revels in one of these forms in particular: seducing the big Subject – as god, master, great men, etc. – while at the same time eluding it.

There is another way out of this structure, but it is more costly: the condition of *psychosis*. Its logic could be formulated as follows: if God *is*, then I *am not*, because being a subject is being sub-jected, in sub-mission, 'placed below'. And to be in sub-mission is not to be, it is to be only by delegation, through an Other. So, God is a god of identity theft, who steals one's very being. The psychotic solution is a radical one, a merciless battle with and against God, which can take two opposite and complementary forms: a paranoid form of persecution by a god who is always attempting to steal my being, who spies on and persecutes me; and a schizophrenic triumphalist form, in which god is... really... me. In both cases, the subject is dealing with a super-natural power, most frequently an imperious voice which occupies the subject in the sense of taking it over and taking possession of it.

This solution is costly because it involves competition with something which is God's prerogative alone, the act of self-foundation. If I am God, I can found myself, just as did the biblical God in his self-referential pronouncement: 'I am who I am.' And indeed, psychotics generally involve God in their delusional states, as the most concentrated expression of the act of self-foundation. The great psychotics like playing equal to God, imitating him, when they are grappling directly with the problem of self-foundation. Countless psychotic narratives deal more or less directly with divine affairs: one day it is a new civilization being born, the next it is a new writing; later it will be a new law or else the steps to be taken to save the world. One need only think of the case of President Schreber or of President Wilson, which Freud analysed so closely. Or equally Artaud, who always claimed that it was him who died on Golgotha 2,000 years previously, and that *he* was God. This structure seems to be able to give new form to what Freud, in one of his last, short but no less crucial texts, calls the *division of the subject* (*Spaltung* in German) (*Die Ichspaltung im Abwehrvorgang*. Freud 1941). We are split beings due to this subjective division, beings who can never really find ourselves because, just when we might be able to do so, we lose ourselves in the big Subject. Lacan, who called this big Subject the Other, capital 'O', worked a lot on this problem, systematically exploring the effects of the repression produced by the confrontation between the little subject and the big Subject.

However, I am also critical of Lacan – which is a way of saying that, unlike some, I do not treat him as a big Subject. My criticism is that he only rarely addresses the specific effects of the big Subject's historical variability. In this respect, Lacan was a man of his time – that is, of structuralism and synchrony to the detriment of diachrony. But the big Subject can only really be perceived in all its complexity if one can grasp and identify its different *avatars*. This is why I have explored the historical figures of the big Subject. I believe that human history is characterized by constant renewal of the figures of the big Subject.

The figures of the big Subject

This renewal is immediately comprehensible in the light of what I stated above, namely that the symbolic remedy for the real affliction of the human being is, at the same time, a poison because I alienate myself in the big Subject. Or, to put it another way, as I said, this big Subject which does not exist, is extremely helpful ... until it becomes extremely cumbersome. So one must kill off one's saviour from time to time, and, after this, reinvent him. And, in fact, when one turns one's attention to historical development, one discovers this big Subject in every imaginable universe constructed by humankind. The big Subject can take the form of a totem, through which a human group chooses an absolute referent in nature. Or else, it can take the form of spirits which inhabit or even haunt places of human habitation. Or of gods immanent to the world who, like the Greek gods of *Physis*, are forever meddling in human affairs. It can also take the form of a transcendent god, an absolute and eternal father, as in the monotheisms. Or it can be incarnated, as in the political religions, in an absolute monarch – as, for example, Louis XIV.

We can assume that this latter big Subject, the absolute monarch, had become a little too big, so, one day, it had to be shortened – this is something we call the French Revolution – with a new big Subject showing up, with, that time, the appearance of the *people*. And we should not forget the political religions of the twentieth century either: Stalinism with its saviour, the proletariat as big Subject, and Nazism with its so-called master race. All of these big Subjects kept alive the symbolic function by constituting a reference point and a foundation for the subject's discourse. But some were, of course, more permanent than others.

Hence, at the heart of our discourses, at the very centre of our culture, of our narratives, can be found one or several discursive beings in which we believe as though these figures were real – be they gods, devils or demons. They represent for the subject, permanence, an origin, an end and an order against the chaos with which he or she is faced. Without this big Subject, this meta-social guarantee, the self is at a loss, does not know where to turn, and the group is likewise endangered, since only a common reference to the same big Subject enables different individuals to feel part of the same community. For the subject, the big Subject is also a foundational point in the past, which makes a temporal order possible; and it is also an exteriority, a 'there', in relation to which an interiority, a 'here', can be formed. In short, for me to be here, I need the big Subject to be there. Without this detour via the big Subject, I am unable to find myself, to accede to the symbolic order, so I am unable to construct space and time for myself. Psychoanalysis, particularly Lacanian psychoanalysis, is a very rich source of understanding on this key issue of access to symbolization. But, as already mentioned, it has remained silent on the issue of the big Subject's historical variation, due to the influence of the prevailing credo of structuralism at the time, it had hypostasised the big Subject in a form valid once and for all, called the Other, capital 'O'. Yet, the big Subject changes constantly with time – or even, history itself is the history of the figures of the big Subject. That is why, some time ago, I started on a research project devoted to historical and geographical variations of the big Subject.

If you agree to suppose, by way of hypothesis, that I have correctly described the big Subject's changing identities and the possibility of its history, then we can immediately see that the distance from myself to what founds me as a subject has got ever shorter. Each of the major stages in the series which goes from the gods (polytheism), to God (monotheism), the king, the republic and the people has brought the big Subject closer to the human universe: we moved from an insurmountable distance between ourselves and the immortals in polytheism, and an infinite distance of transcendence in the monotheisms, to the throne, halfway between Heaven and Earth in monarchy, and then to the intra-worldly separation of the individual and the collective in the republic. The distance between the subject and the big Subject has, each time, been reduced. This is not a continuous progression, of course, and there have been all sorts of movements, back and forth, and aberrations like race, but still the principle holds.

At this point I am able to suggest a definition of modernity. If pre-modernity was the space in which the subject was subjected to *one* figure of the big Subject, modernity is the space in which the subject is defined by *several* of these occurrences of the big Subject. Modernity arrives when the world ceases to be closed and becomes, as Alexandre Koyré has shown, open, or even 'infinite' – in its symbolic references also (Koyré 1957). Modernity is this space in which subjects are subjected to gods, God, the king, the republic, the people. All of these figures can be found in modernity, which likes nothing better than to change from one to the other. This explains the mobile, 'crisisful' and critical aspect of modernity. In modernity, the ultimate referent changes all the time, and hence symbolic space as a whole becomes mobile. Modernity is thus inhabited by Otherness, indeed by many big Subjects, or figures of the big Subject. That is why the subjective condition in modernity can be defined by a further feature, in addition to that of *neurosis* mentioned above concerning primary processes, namely *criticism* concerning secondary processes. This *critical* approach derives from the fact that the subject of modernity plays on several references at once, which are in competition or even in conflict with each other. This is of decisive importance for the institutions of modernity. As institutions interpellating and producing modern subjects, they can exist only as spaces defined by *critical* thinking. Reason, the reason of the Enlightenment, can be redefined as a space opened in thought, in which all possible disagreements on the great referents of the past, the present and the future are debated *ad infinitum*. In short, the modern subject is, as a subject, *neurotic* and, as a modern subject, *critical*.

Post-modern subjectivity

You may remember that almost 40 years ago, in 1979 to be precise, the philosopher J.-F. Lyotard claimed that a break had occurred in modernity. In his remarkable and bold book entitled *The Postmodern Condition* (Lyotard 1984), significantly published a year before the ultraliberals came to power in two of the most important countries in the world, United Kingdom (Thatcher) and the USA (Reagan), Lyotard noted that, with the exhaustion and disappearance of grand foundational narratives, we were exiting from modernity and entering a 'post-modern' era. Lyotard described our new condition in the following terms: we were leaving behind the grand theo-logico-political narratives, both the ancient ones (like monotheisms) and the modern ones (I mean the narratives of *individual emancipation* through access to critical rationality and those of *collective emancipation* – as in Marxism, for example). Now the collapse of these grand narratives is also the collapse of the figures of the big Subject which these narratives sustained. The basic structures of our world have been overturned by post-modernity. And this inevitably implies a radical transformation of our subjective condition. I mean that being a subject is significantly different today, in our democratic market economies, from what it was in past generations. In short, I am inclined to believe that today's subject is altogether different from the subject which existed only one or two generations ago. And since our subjective condition varies historically, we can surmise that we have just entered a new phase which particularly affects our major institutions producing the subjects, such as the family, schools, health care, mental health and justice.

That is why, after evoking the different figures of the big Subject, I must now evoke its decline and disappearance. We might find the destruction of idols interesting, but we should not neglect the serious problems this poses. Post-modernity has no other presentable figures of the big Subject to propose. While the preceding periods were defined by the (greater or lesser) distance of the subject to what founds it, post-modernity can be defined as the abolition of the distance between the subject and the big Subject. You might point out that this collapse of the big Subject is nothing to worry about because we now have the Market. But I have a great many doubts about the capacity of what we call 'the market' to embody a new big Subject. It does not function as a grand collective narrative, but as an infinity of small ego-oriented ones. Which is why, even if it is often presented as the cure to all our ills, it is utterly inadequate as a new big Subject because it can never respond to the question of the origin. Rather, it confronts each of us with the torments (which, of course, do not exclude certain pleasures) of self-foundation. The basic, fundamental limit of the market economy in its claim to cover the whole field of social and personal bonds is that the market is not a general economy, not a symbolic economy either, but simply an 'economic economy': an economic economy based on a libidinal economy insofar as it is a constant source of manufactured objects supposed to satisfy our every desire, but it fails to function as a general economy because it has nothing to offer the subject on the problem of foundation. In post-modernity, the subject is no longer defined by its dependence on God, the king or the republic, but only by itself. This is why there is so much talk of individualism.

Two of the many implications of this new definition of the subject are its legal autonomy and its economic freedom. In liberal theory, as you know, economic freedom is the very cornerstone of capitalism. We must be free to pursue our egotistical interests because, through these, society's collective interests are assured – as they say. Today, we thus have a configuration of legal autonomy, market freedom – which can be total freedom, as in today's neoliberalism – and a self-referential definition of the speaking subject. So today we are free, but, in contrast to what we might have expected, we are probably going to have to pay a very high price for this. This freedom, this Enlightenment ideal, which we have managed to wrest from subservience to idols, could ultimately prove extremely costly to us. What I wish to draw attention to is that the subject is defined, here, self-referentially. The subject no longer points to a big Subject as founding the subject. And when there are no longer any big Subjects, the problems start. Why? Because just when subjects in general are commanded to be nothing but themselves, being oneself becomes the most difficult, or even impossible, task. This explains why our post-modern societies increasingly have recourse to techniques for acting on the self, from television programmes which stage people's everyday lives, to mind-altering drugs for boosting one's morale and unleashing one's potential. With post-modernity, what was once the distance from oneself to the big Subject has become a distance within oneself. Every subject thus has to get to grips with its own self-foundation, and it can certainly succeed – but not without encountering serious failures. Distance is thus discovered to be internal and, moreover, inherent to the post-modern subject, and this significantly modifies Freud's diagnosis of the modern subject and its tendency to neurosis. The subjective condition of the post-modern subject can be defined, rather, as a tendency towards a borderline state between neurosis and psychosis, like narcissistic psychoneuroses, increasingly caught between a latent melancholy (the famous 'depression'), the inability to speak in the first person, the illusion of omnipotence and repeated evasions in the form of false selves or multiple personalities, available in all shapes and sizes on the cultural market.

In post-modernity, the subject is no longer defined by neurotic guilt, but rather by the feeling of omnipotence when he succeeds, and of total impotence when he does not. The symbolic universe of the post-modern subject is not that of the modern subject: without a big Subject – that is, without a marker by which symbolic anteriority and exteriority may be grounded – the subject is unable to create for itself sufficiently broad spatial and temporal coordinates. It remains fixed in a present which is its only dimension. Some scholars call that *presentism*. The relation to others becomes problematic insofar as personal survival is constantly at stake. If everything is at stake all the time, then plans, anticipation and self-questioning become very difficult operations. The whole universe of critique is thus undermined. The subject as consumer replaces the critical subject.

How to respond to this absence of the big Subject? One solution is to construct oneself all alone, using all the many resources of our so-called information societies. We witness an increasing number of people who have trodden unusual educational pathways. The subject educates him- or herself, using all the material and human resources available, with sometimes spectacular results. This is due to the fact that we have autonomy where previously there was heteronomy. But this autonomy, which is given to us immediately, and no longer at the end of a long process, is what also confronts individuals with the greatest difficulty: that of being themselves. Today, people can easily fall prey to whatever seems to satisfy their immediate needs. Post-modern subjects are thus easy targets for that immensely powerful apparatus called the market, which can entirely overrun people's lives and take control of everything, due to its capacity to affect and dominate our daily time (particularly through TV, film, games, ads, etc. more and more disseminated by new and individual technologies). The docility with which many adolescents wear and exhibit brand name clothing is a sign of this new servitude, which may well be involuntary, but which is no less real for all that. This shows, I believe, that we have moved from a mostly symbolic to a mostly libidinal functioning. What, after all, does the market do, if not offer – I mean sell – to the subject who is grappling with his or her internal difficulties, a manufactured object, a paying service or a tailor-made phantasm produced by the culture industries, and which claims that it satisfies all our drives and desires?

It goes beyond the scope of this chapter to show how the disappearance of grand narratives and of the figures of the big Subject go hand in hand with the end of ideology, the disappearance of the avant-gardes, the development of egoism, the shrinkage of the state, the increasing value placed on commodities and consumerism beyond all other considerations, the decisive rule of having money, the transformation of culture into changing fashions, the homogenization of ways of life at the same time as their individualization and the exhibitionist display of surface signs, the flattening-out of history, leaving nothing but the immediacy of the event and snapshots of information, the central place taken by extremely powerful and frequently uncontrolled technologies, the unravelling of the institution of the family, the intense questioning of sexual identity, the public exhibition of private space and the privatization of public space – and so forth. All these features should be read as significant symptoms of this passage from modern to post-modern culture – that is, to the culture of the neoliberal era.

Lastly, let me say that having renounced the fiction of the big Subject we may well have freed ourselves from the old tyrannical idols, but we are also faced with 'impossible' questions for which 'the Market' provides no answers. I hope this approach could help to understand some important changes from modern to post-modern subjectivities and pathologies.

Ways of compensating for the absence of the big Subject

Some subjects feel bereft of the big Subject and seek as best they can to compensate for its absence. I have identified five compensating strategies, five ways which are perfectly 'logical'. These strategies seem to me to be practised especially by a great many adolescents and young adults in our post-modern societies: addiction (to replace the big Subject in the order not of a symbolic desire but of real need), groups and gangs (to support with other small subjects the absence of the big Subject), sects and fundamentalisms (to provide a new big Subject more powerful than old big Subjects) and research of omnipotence (where somebody feels invested with the big Subject's omnipotence). All these strategies constitute extremely serious problems for education and health professionals.

First, *dependence or addiction*. When the big Subject is lacking, one can try to reinscribe it in the order not of desire but of need. Consumer products can play this role, and we witness fully fledged addictions to these. There is one in particular which has the terrifying privilege of being illegal, rare and expensive, and hence much more tempting than the others, namely drugs. Through drug use we can reinscribe the big Subject in the order not of desire but of need. In drug dependency, the issue is no longer turning the difficulty of existence into a symbolic quest in which artistic creations (poems, dance, singing, music, painting) must be carefully constructed and expressed in order to supplement the usual imperfections of the big Subject. With drug addiction, this laborious quest is transformed into a simple dependence on the big Subject, who no longer operates in the field of desire, but, I repeat, is in a sense reinscribed into the real of need. At least in that way, the big Subject, whose lack we feel, can be known and located, in the form of a chemical product which is as addictive as possible, and which we can have access to, on condition that we become its slave. We know the devastating effects of intensive (rather than occasional) drug use.

Second, *groups and gangs*. When the big Subject is lacking and one is incapable of taking up the challenges of autonomy or self-foundation on one's own, one can always try to do so alongside others. All one has to do is belong to a single entity made up of several distinct parts. This is what one calls a group in the sense of gang. Groups are characterized by transitivism – that is, all group members are part of the same person, such that if one of them falls over, the others feel pain. The group has a collective name displayed by each member for all to see; it has a signature, an acronym and a tag, which stakes out the limits of its territory – one need only take the train to see the extent of this phenomenon. If an individual happens to dissociate him- or herself from the collective personality figured by the group – for example, by taking an interest in something other than what the group is interested in – the group, which jealously cannot bear one of its members breaking away, feels obliged to reclaim the individual by all possible means. So it is sometimes almost impossible for a school teacher to address a *single* pupil belonging to a group because it is the whole group which comes forward and responds to the slightest remark, displaying its prerogatives and objects. We are in the fusion of all individuals into a single entity, preferably embodied in the group's leader. A variant on the group is the gang. It is in some sense the natural extension of the group. The gang is a group which has become successful by imposing its summary methods such as rackets, assault, the settling of scores and so forth. In schools in disadvantaged areas groups are particularly prone to transforming into gangs.

Third, *sects*. When the big Subject is lacking, one can do one's utmost to erect a sort of big Subject which will provide an absolute guarantee against the experience of absence. This is what we see in the many sects which flourish in our post-modern societies – a little group gets together, brandishes the image of a guru or of the newest absolute master, or of a vengeful god. And clearly, in our globalized age, this phenomenon, with the fundamentalisms we see around us, can have a worldwide impact.

Fourth, *omnipotence*. Another way in which we can dispense with the absent big Subject is if we are able to consider ourselves invested with the big Subject's omnipotence. In self-infatuation, the self-referential movement previously attached to the big Subject has migrated to the little subject. This results in perversion, in which individuals seek to instrumentalize others and, in extreme cases, to appropriate for themselves the power of life and death over their fellow creatures, imagining themselves to be endowed with magical powers. This move is abetted today by the social prestige of the techno-sciences, which constantly supply us with more powerful prostheses, thus bolstering our sense of omnipotence. We hear of the most brutal acts of violence on a daily basis. We hear of the most brutal acts of violence on a daily basis. Shootings and killings have been occurring regularly, particularly in schools – and the phenomenon even seems to be on the increase.

Finally, there is a fifth tendency, when none of the above seem to work – and that is the solution of *depression*. As I mentioned above, it is when one is commanded to be oneself that one encounters the greatest difficulty precisely in being oneself. In depression, one can no longer believe in oneself. One becomes less than oneself. It is said that over a quarter of us go through more or less severe phases of depression.

Why did they do it?

There is no reason to think that these different strategies could not go together: it is possible to be a member of a group or a gang, drug-dependent, a member of a fundamentalist sect and extremely violent. Recent examples of such convergence are, of course, the 'terrorist attacks' in Paris and Brussels. Much has already been written and said about these, but something might be added in the light of the theme discussed in this chapter: the absence of the Big Subject. I will focus here a moment on the historical context of the Paris massacres.

My children, my students, they have asked me: 'But why did they do it?'. I refer my upset enquirers to the excellent interview with my colleague and friend, psychoanalyst Fethi Benslama, which appeared in the major press 24 hours before the horror. He said – and here we have his premonitory intelligence – 'for the desperate, radical Islamism is an exciting thing'.[1] He explained that youngsters who are distressed due to important identity flaws are charmed by the jihadist offer because it provides them with an absolute ideal that fills up these flaws. It is an offer that transforms the subject fallen prey to torments of foundation into a 'fanatical automaton'. Benslama's article is not an occasional text. It springs from research work undertaken since the years in which the clinical view found itself enriched by anthropological, historical and philosophical approaches regarding the understanding and clarification of the subjectivation modes arising from the Arab-Muslim culture. On 13 November many readers who watched television and discovered the horror, and I was one of them, had the odd impression of having read the day before, in the paper of the 12th, the news of the next day – like in a disquieting remake of René Clair's movie *C'est arrivé demain*, 'It has happened tomorrow'. Of course, nothing mediumistic was going on there. Fethi Benslama contents himself with being a clinician. An extremely sensible clinician, however, since he was able to produce what today seems like a perfect 'clinical photofit' of the exterminators.

Fethi Benslama traces the mentioned identity flaw back to the fall of the last Caliphate (1924), which embodied the principle of theologico-political sovereignty in Islam. This principle, that did not separate the temporal from the spiritual, nor, a fortiori, the state from religion, utilizes the *sharia* (the Koranic law) to regulate the totality of the life of the believer. The Caliph being the successor of Mohammed, the fall of the Caliphate produced an enormous trauma because the direct lineage with the Prophet, which had maintained itself from one Caliphate to the other over 1,400 years, was now broken. While the Ottoman territory was split up on behalf of colonial powers – that is France and England – the first lay state was born in Turkey. The Muslims have thus passed from a position of being their own master to that of subordinate, while losing the direct link with God and being abruptly thrown into modernity. Not surprisingly then, shortly after that ruin, in 1928, the Muslim Brotherhood appeared, promising the restoration of the Caliphate and the dismantlement of the new states. They were the first of a whole series of ever more radical Islamist groups.

That was, for certain, a major flaw. However, it seems to me to have been worsened by other flaws. There is one, much earlier, which goes back to the difficulties Islam (that until the Middle Ages had contributed so much to civilization) had with taking the turn of the Enlightenment, which implicates not only the separation of the temporal and the spiritual, but also the possible assumption of a subject thinking and acting by himself.

And there were other flaws, later. Like the vote of the United Nations in 1947 which split Palestine into a Jewish state and a Arab state that has never been established, an omission which has provoked a chain of reciprocal reprisals seizing the whole region of the Middle East and beyond. Like the colonial war France waged against Algeria, framed by two massacres: that of Sétif in May 1945, with about 10,000 Algerian casualties, and that of 17 October 1961 in Paris, when about 100 Algerian demonstrators were thrown into the Seine from the bridges of Neuilly, Argenteuil and Asnières. In between these two massacres was an endless cycle of vindictive violence unleashed with its share of outrage (executions, violations, attacks, generalization of torture). Balance: about 500,000 killed, of which 400,000 Algerians, 4,000 *pieds noirs*, 30,000 French and 20,000 Harki soldiers. Like the invasion in 2003 of a large Arab state, Iraq, by a coalition led by the USA. If we need to examine this, it is because the twenty-first century has not finished yet paying the price for the decision George W. Bush made to hold Saddam Hussein responsible for the destruction on 11 September 2001 of one of the symbols of American power, the twin towers of the World Trade Center in Manhattan. In other words, the century opened with a capital mistake – if it were not a monstrous strategic manipulation, which will produce a parade of catastrophic after-effects.

A brief recapitulation of the facts: 1) certainly Saddam was a dictator, of the same sort, by the way, as the ones that Washington has always supported (for example, Pinochet), but he had nothing to do with that destruction (the American intelligence knew that he did not maintain ties with Al-Qaeda); 2) the Bushian promise, echoed – among others – by Tony Blair, to bring democracy to Iraq (the operation was called 'Iraqi Freedom') was nothing but a slogan used to win over the western public opinion; 3) the proof put forward to destroy Saddam's regime was nothing but a collection of glaring mistakes (for instance, the famous 'weapons of mass destruction', which were never found). In fact, what was at stake here was an all too transparent narrative assembly (deserving the title of worst kind of storytelling management), with the aim of getting hold of the fourth largest global oil reserve. This was not a coincidence: Bush himself and a large part of his government are, it is known, closely linked to the oil industry.

Today we know what the catastrophic geo-strategic outcomes were of this intervention: at least 500,000 Iraqis killed, a mortality rate that went up from 5.5 per 1,000 before the invasion to 13.2 after the arrival of the Americans, a disastrous sanitary balance (80 per cent of the water henceforth is untreated), a devastated country fallen prey to religious battles from other days and, above all, a laboratory for the formation of jihadist militias who dream of reinstating the Caliphate, regimenting all forms of human life and making millions of 'normal' people take flight. They thrive in countries at war like Syria, welcoming, training and transforming into belligerent terrorists thousands of young people coming from Europe and elsewhere, suffering from the identity flaw brought up by Fethi Benslama.

It has been the honour of France not to let itself get caught up in such a disastrous enterprise, in spite of strong appeals by 'intellectuals' who presently find themselves in agreement with the Front National in denouncing migrants, the enormous floods of which result directly from the war they have supported. The day after the American invasion they were so bold to publish a 'viewpoint' that started with these surrealist lines: 'What a joy to see the Iraqi people in an elated mood celebrating their liberation and … their liberators!'[2] Fortunately sensible political people did not go along with them. One will recollect for a long time the speech President Chirac's Minister of Foreign Affairs, Dominique de Villepin, gave at the United Nations on 14 February 2003, in which he said that France would not join that coalition because, and I quote: 'Such an intervention threatens to worsen the fractures between societies, between cultures, between people, fractures on which terrorism feeds.'[3]

The question poses itself, then, how France, which saw things correctly (thereby arousing the persistent wrath of Republican Americans, so-called hawks who could better be called asses[4]), has become one of the most important targets of jihadism. The answer to that becomes perfectly clear if one does not forget about history: we have moved from a Gaullian to an Atlanticist position. The Gaullian view was not really called into question by Mitterand and was passed on up to Chirac. The latter understood at least two things very well: an external principle: no bond with Washington; and an internal principle: the French state has to reckon with the fact that about 10 per cent of its residents is of Arab origin. This strategic principle and this pragmatic principle account for the good relations Chirac had with Arab leaders. Sarkozy's coming to power was marked by an Atlanticist turn suggesting indecency when one thinks of the docile loyalty declared to Bush. In practice, this expressed itself by the reintegration of France into command of the North Atlantic Treaty Organization. De Gaulle had announced France's withdrawal from NATO on 21 February 1966. Sarkozy went to Washington – or to Canossa – himself on 7 November 2007, to announce its return. And his successor, François Hollande, has done nothing to change the direction of this Atlanticist course. On the contrary, the French government henceforth surpassed the American administration in the defence of Israeli politics, notwithstanding the considerable dimensions of the colonies which segmented Palestinian territory. A coarse strategy, so unlike the intelligence of the Jews who have always managed to live among others, to obstruct the formation of a Palestinian state which yet was explicitly intended by international resolutions. Why did France start to bomb the neighbouring country of Iraq, Syria, in September 2015? Why did it not let the Americans account for the consequences of their disastrous politics in Iraq and neighbouring countries? For these foolish politicians have created a monster, the jihadis: these automatons without discernment, without thought, without human feelings.[5]

So, after the attack on Charlie Hebdo, Hollande must have been happily playing his part in reinforcing considerably the security of the country and the population. But he wanted more than that: to become master of war. It was not the first time one could see a head of state, troubled by a waning popularity, picking, consciously or not, the option of war in hopes of getting the support of the people. Be that as it may, Hollande thought he was fighting a distant war, but it is here. This double Atlanticist turn has contributed in no small measure to making France – our beloved Paris of the Revolution, of the Commune, of the Liberation, of May 1968 – our youth, my children, my students, who love life, thought, love, feast, the laughter of Charlie or the rock of Bataclan – henceforth directly targeted.

All this can be summarized in one sentence: the jihadists in the sphere of influence of the Islamic State of Iraq and Syria (ISIS) are, like the Nazis of yesteryear, dangerous lunatics, but some prominent western executives have substantially contributed to them becoming such. These psychopaths are products of our so-called free world and they are keeping a lethal delirium going; nobody knows when it might end. They turned up, after all, as the offspring of fathers who have been excluded, humiliated, one could say humiliated quadruply: the fall of the Caliphate, Palestine, Algeria, Iraq. Here they are, in the position of sub-Muslims, dreaming about nothing other than avenging the Father by making themselves into super-Muslims (the term comes from Fethi Benslama and evokes the formation of a ferocious and obscene super-ego). The road to pass from one state to the other is simple: to die. Dying while killing as many 'infidels' as possible becomes, for them, the complete fulfilment. In this way they can transform a life which is worthless to them and in which they are nothing but unworthy outcasts into a life in which they are everything, since the martyr in Islam is a death that stays alive, and even more than alive: immortal. Dying in these circumstances opens the gate for them to Paradise, where they will enjoy a superior life, recompensed by the *houris* (the virgins spoken of in Surah 55, verse 56) who await them. What can be done against a delirium that eroticizes death like this, or, even more, that makes death into a supreme orgasm? It takes the lucidity of a laical Arab writer like Kamel Daoud to dare to think that what is at stake here probably is the direct counterpart of the fact that 'sex is the largest misery in the world of Allah'.[6]

To return, finally, to the theme of this chapter: regarding the absence of the big Subject or the Other one can notice the rising of a sentiment of omnipotence in individuals who believe that they have become the almighty Other themselves. In extreme cases these super-individuals may take the liberty of deciding about life and death of their fellow men, equipping themselves ever more easily with magical powers because of the contribution of the techno-sciences in stirring up feelings of omnipotence (e.g. GoPro cameras, sophisticated arms, digital image and sound technology, the possibility to address the whole world via the internet). Acts of most extreme violence thus can erupt in an unbridled way. One has lost count of the violent outbursts which, in the West, fill the news. The Paris massacres can be placed within a series of crimes which have spread through the West since the start of neoliberalism. They go from the crime of Corporal Lortie in the National Assembly of Quebec in 1984 to the killings at Sandy Hook in the United States in 2012, with dozens of other shootings in between. They all arise from the same delirious calculation: if the Other is no more, I have to become the Other. In other words: the Other, that is me. Or again: I will replace the Other eliminated by post-modernity with an Other coming from pre-modernity.

Notes

1 www.lemonde.fr/societe/article/2015/11/12/pour-les-desesperes-l-islamisme-radical-est-un-produit-excitant_4808430_3224.html (accessed 21 June 2016).
2 http://www.lemonde.fr/international/article/2003/04/14/point-de-vue-la-faute-par-pascal-bruckner-andre-glucksmann-et-romain-goupil_316794_3210.html (accessed 21 June 2016).
3 http://www.lefigaro.fr/politique/le-scan/2014/04/08/25001-20140408 ARTFIG00066-le-discours-de-villepin-sur-l-irak-a-l-onu.php (accessed 21 June 2016).
4 Dufour's wordplay here is *faucon* (hawk) versus *neo-con* (neo-con[servative] *and* neo-prick).
5 See the excellent novel *2084* by Sansal Boualem (2015).
6 See the very courageous opinion piece by the Algerian author in *Le Monde* of 31 January 2016: 'Cologne, place of phantasms' (where, during New Year's Eve 2016, more than 1,000 violations of a sexual nature were committed against women by men described as North-African or Arab). Being lucid is not a good thing: a fatwa was issued against Kamel Daoud by a salaphist imam who called out for his execution. http://www.lemonde.fr/idees/article/2016/01/31/cologne-lieu-de-fantasmes_4856694_3232.html (accessed 21 June 2016).

References

Aristotle (1966): *The Works of Aristotle*, ed. W.D. Ross. Oxford: Oxford University Press.
Boualem, S. (2015): *2084. La Fin du Monde*. Paris: Gallimard.
Dufour, D.-R. (1999): *Lettres sur la nature humaine à l'usage des survivants*. Paris: Calmann-Lévy.
Dufour, D.-R. (2005): *On achéve bien les hommes. De quelques conséquences actuelles et futures de la mort de Dieu*. Paris: Denoël.
Dufour, D.-R. (2012): *Il était une fois le dernier homme*. Paris: Denoël.
Freud, S. (1941): *Gesammelte Werke*, Bd. 17. London: Imago.
Freud, S. (1948/1926): *Gesammelte Werke*, Bd. 14. London: Imago.
Koyré, A. (1957): *From the Closed World to the Infinite Universe*. Baltimore, MD: Johns Hopkins University Press.
Lacan, J. (1992): *The Seminar of Jacques Lacan. Book VII: The Ethics of Psychoanalysis*. New York/London: Routledge.
Lyotard, J.-F. (1984): *The Postmodern Condition: A Report on Knowledge*. Manchester: Manchester University Press.

3 Return of the age of anxiety

The embedding of a late modern social pathology

Anders Petersen

Introduction

According to Ulrich Beck and Wolfgang Bonss (2001: 63), one of the fundamental tasks of sociology is diagnosis of the times.[1] Actually, one can make the claim that sociology – on an overall level – has always had the ambition to try to diagnose the essential character of society (Lichtblau 1995). That claim is not hard to support. One just has to direct attention towards the analysis of the founding fathers of the discipline, more specifically their analysis of the transition from traditional to modern society. Marx, Simmel, Durkheim and Weber – they all focused on the consequences of this rupture and the malaises it brought about: anomie, alienation, rational iron cage and tragedy of culture. In relation to the diagnosis of contemporary society, the concepts and analyses of the founding fathers are no longer adequate. We have, as so many authors have reported, moved on to a new historical epoch. A wide range of names has been given to this epoch – post-modernity (Lyotard 1979); hypermodernity (Lipovetsky 2005); liquid modernity (Bauman 2000) and late modernity (Giddens 1991) – just to mention a few. Whatever conceptualization one prefers, the concepts used to capture the essential character of this epoch have changed and so have the malaises that encapsulate our particular age.[2]

Which malaise, then, is indicative of our historical epoch? A bit more than a decade ago, American sociologist Allan V. Horwitz and American Philosopher Jerome Wakefield tried to capture this in their article 'The age of depression' (Horwitz and Wakefield 2005). The starting point of their article is actually that we have witnessed a transformation from the age of anxiety to the age of depression. But why?[3] Their main claim is simply that depression is to be perceived as the pivotal mental disorder that informs us in the best possible way about the conditions of living in contemporary society because of two factors: first of all, western countries have witnessed a swelling prevalence in the amount of people who have been diagnosed with depression; second, a steep increase in the amount of people on antidepressant medication has been detected. The argumentation in the article is solid and the claims are well substantiated.[4] However, a shift seems to be occurring. And although depression is still a significant (and troubling) mental disorder in contemporary society, it appears to have been overtaken by another mental disorder, namely anxiety. Perhaps one can even talk about a comeback of anxiety?

In 1947 (first in New York – then in 1948 in London) W.H. Auden famously proclaimed that time to be 'the age of anxiety' (Auden 1948). In his lengthy poem Auden, in the form of a dramatic allegory, identifies – and manifests – the basic human problem as man's anxiety in time. Written in the aftermath of World War II, one understands why Auden's poem is permeated with pessimism – especially concerning the psychic condition of his contemporaries. As Edward Callan writes:

> The plot of *The Age of Anxiety* reveals, not character development in the conventional sense, but development within the psychic personality. More specifically, the six parts of *The Age of Anxiety* are six stages in a regenerative journey; and, furthermore, each of the four central acts of the drama presents a search for 'Wholeness'.
>
> Callan 1965: 157

The Age of Anxiety, in Callan's interpretation, thus voices a growing psychic fragmentation. There is a lack of wholeness at stake that is creating immense individual difficulties. People are torn apart and in desperate need of completeness. But alas – their search seems to be in vain. Now, the question arises whether Auden's description of the age of anxiety is adequate when it comes to the age of anxiety that we are witnessing now. I think not. By answering in the negative, I am not questioning whether we in fact live in an age of anxiety. Because I – alongside many others (for example, Wilkinson 2001; Parish 2001; Salecl 2004; Horwitz 2013) – think that we do. I simply believe that we need another vocabulary to capture the specificities of this age rather than the one provided by Auden. In other words: I want to avoid the risk of portraying anxiety as a historical constant, however comforting that might be. Hence, in this chapter I will present the outline of an analysis that tries to answer one main question: why is anxiety indicative of our time?

In order to answer this question in an acceptable manner I will proceed in four stages. First, I will substantiate the main claim of the article and explicate how one can legitimately call our age the age of anxiety. Second, I will elucidate specific kind(s) of anxiety that are sweeping through contemporary western societies and discuss why these kinds are particularly actualized. Third, I will explain why these kinds of anxiety (the kinds that seem to be very prevalent among youth and adolescence) are to be understood as signs of social pathology and not just individualized disorders. Fourth, I will conclude by discussing the main points of the chapter and by elaborating on future research possibilities that the chapter enables.

Why the age of anxiety?

So far I have – in an unhesitant way – addressed anxiety as a particular mental disorder. To most contemporaries, I would claim, this is rather unproblematic.

But that has not always been the case. When Søren Kierkegaard embarked on his famous philosophical/psychological (in fact, Kierkegaard called himself a psychologist when writing *On the Concept of Anxiety*, not a philosopher) journey into the concept of anxiety, no mention of anxiety as mental disorder came to mind. Instead, anxiety to Kierkegaard was to be perceived as an existential and religious (strongly connected with hereditary sin) embedded condition, which individuals had to address when making free choices. Thus, according to Kierkegaard, anxiety was intrinsically linked with freedom. As he writes:

> Anxiety may be compared with dizziness. He whose eye happens to look down into the yawning abyss becomes dizzy. But what is the reason for this? It is just as much in his own eye as in the abyss, for suppose he had not looked down. Hence anxiety is the dizziness of freedom, which emerges when the spirit wants to posit the synthesis and freedom looks down into its own possibility, laying hold of finiteness to support itself.
>
> Kierkegaard 1980: 61

There is quite a long way from this Kierkegaardian perspective on anxiety to mental disorder. The same is true if we move towards cultural understandings of anxiety that reigned in the past. As Allan V. Horwitz writes: 'Through much of the twentieth century, anxiety was not only a central condition in medical and psychiatric practice but also a major aspect of Western culture' (Horwitz 2013: 118). In fact, for most of this century anxiety was not even formulated as a disease. The cultural aspect of anxiety took precedence over the medical, one could say. According to Horwitz, three major influences can explain this.

First of all, Sigmund Freud's pathbreaking theoretical perspective on anxiety was immensely popular among intellectuals and in the media. In Freud's earlier writings, more specifically in 1894, he coined the term 'anxiety neurosis' (Freud 1959/1926). According to Freud, this form of neurosis was a distinct syndrome with distinct symptoms, which were quite different from those of neurasthenia. At that time, neurasthenia was a very popular and successful diagnosis, a nosology instituted by American neurologist George Miller Beard in 1869. The overall reason why neurasthenia – or nervous exhaustion (Beard 1869) – enjoyed such immense popularity[5] was due to the fact that it described an illness of modern life – increased nervous exhaustion brought about by the emergence of modern industries and big cities. Hence, the aetiology of neurasthenia was to be found in the social permeability of the mind rather than in biomedical alterations of the brain. The problem with the term 'neurasthenia', however, was its scope. It encompassed everything. As Beard wrote:

> If a patient complains of general malaise, debility of all the functions, poor appetite, abiding weakness in the back and spine, fugitive neuralgic pains, hysteria, insomnia, hypochondriasis, disinclination for consecutive mental labour, severe and weakening attack of sick headache, and other analogous

symptoms, and at the same time gives no evidence of anaemia or any organic disease, we have reason to suspect... that we are dealing with a typical case of neurasthenia.

Beard, in Ehrenberg 2010b: 32

Freud was dissatisfied with this, and extracted the anxiety neurosis as a particular syndrome from neurasthenia. He grouped a whole range of symptoms and identified them as having different manifestations – heart and breathing problems, panic, psychic obsessions etc. – of the same underlying process. In Freud's interpretation, anxiety neurosis was (and so was neurasthenia) the result of sexual dissatisfaction, and it ultimately 'stemmed from the accumulation of more sexual excitation than people could psychically assimilate. Anxiety neurosis were thus especially common among sexually frustrated practitioners of *coitus interruptus*, sexual abstinence, and the like' (Horwitz 2013: 79). In that respect, anxiety neuroses was more a synonym for culturally imbued distress than for a particular mental disease.

Second, anxiety played (and still plays) a major role in existential philosophy, which – generally speaking – addressed anxiety as a core human predicament. Just think of the writings of existential philosophers Jean-Paul Sartre, Martin Heidegger and Martin Buber, whose thoughts and ideas were highly popular and manifested themselves in the cultural landscape of the twentieth century. Of course, the proliferation of their ideas about anxiety did not strike a chord with the vast majority of the western population. But the idea, nevertheless, that anxiety was an inherent part of human life – and that socio-cultural transformations could alter the particular manifestations of anxiety – became axiomatic. Understood as such, anxiety was not to be seen as a medical condition.

Third, it was commonplace in especially the middle of the twentieth century to perceive anxiety as a natural response to socially and politically generated circumstances. In the post-war period – precipitated by the horrific experiences of Holocaust and Hiroshima – anxiety arose in the face of catastrophic tensions of the cold war, the proliferation of nuclear weapons and uncertainties of the geopolitical situation per se. The greatest hostilities between the USA and the former Communist states are emblematic of this reception of anxiety. One of the central characteristics of the political climate of the time is how anxiety was directly related to something that came from the outside and potentially invaded – and thus disrupted and manipulated – the entire social body. Images of parasites and bacteria were used to delineate how the 'others' could colonize every pore of society. The feeling of anxiety was, undoubtedly, heightened by these circumstances. But there was something that further stimulated this, namely specific societal developments. As Slovenian philosopher Renata Salecl writes: 'And then, too, economic crisis became coupled with the crisis of man trying to figure out the idea of the future' (Salecl 2004: 2). Still, however, anxiety in this guise is not to be mistaken for a specific medical condition or disease: it was a socio-cultural signifier.

All of this has changed. Nowadays, anxiety is mostly perceived as a mental disorder with crippling individual consequences. In order to understand why this has become the case, one cannot avoid dealing with the transformation of the discipline of psychiatry. As historian Edward Shorter has argued, the discipline of psychiatry has – almost since its birth – been biologically/medically oriented. That is, with one major exception, namely what he refers to as the psychoanalytic hiatus (Shorter 1997: 145). In relation to this chapter, this hiatus is of great importance since it directly refers to the period of time when anxiety was not necessarily perceived to be a medical disorder in need of treatment. As already mentioned, Freud, as well as his contemporary followers, reserved another place for anxiety than the strictly medical. But the Freudian perspective did not last long, which Shorter's final chapter in his history of psychiatry also indicates: the chapter is entitled From 'Freud to Prozac' (ibid.: 288). Thus, at some point the medical perspective on anxiety gained prominence, something that actually can be dated to the publication of the *DSM-III* in 1980. The launch of this version of the *DSM* announced what Allan V. Horwitz has called a transformation from dynamic to diagnostic psychiatry (Horwitz 2002). In the *DSM-III* all psychoanalytic analysis, language and jargon was removed, thereby altering the focus of psychiatric enquiry. As Horwitz writes:

> In contrast to the dynamic model, diagnostic psychiatry defines diseases through the presence of overt symptoms, regardless of the causes of these symptoms. It regards diseases as natural entities that exist in the body and that generate the particular symptoms a person displays. These diseases became the object of scientific claims that can be made in isolation from the personalities and social contexts in which they arise, an abstraction that would have been unthinkable in the dynamic model.
>
> Ibid.: 56–7

Within the realm of diagnostic psychiatry, the primary causes of mental disorders are not sought in childhood disturbances – or in difficult socio-economic living conditions for that matter – but in disturbed brains and neurochemical activities, all of which manifests itself in various symptoms that can be observed and communicated. In that respect the main focus is on symptoms that can be classified and collected into a given diagnosis. What is particularly interesting in this transition is, of course, the ways in which anxiety was imbedded in this new philosophy. Horwitz again: 'The *DSM-III* revolutionized conceptions of anxiety' (Horwitz 2013: 134). First of all, the *DSM-III* separated anxiety from depression and hence chose to distinguish sharply between those two malaises – something which Edward Shorter has problematized (Shorter 2013). Second, and this is what Horwitz primarily refers to, the *DSM-III* initiated a complete societal implementation of anxiety as a medical, and hence diagnosable, disease that can be treated with pharmaceuticals – first and foremost antidepressants. Due to this development, other languages of anxiety than the diagnostic have, gradually, been replaced. In that respect, the dominant medical language of anxiety is an intrinsic part of what I have elsewhere referred to as the diagnostic culture (Brinkmann and Petersen 2015). The main characteristic of the diagnostic culture is the fact that psychological problems, human deviance and malaises are predominantly understood as something that can be diagnosed on the grounds of its various symptoms. Hence, anxiety is no longer – by laymen as well as medical professionals – addressed as a moral, ethical, existential or even psychological problem but as a set of symptoms indicative of a medical disorder that needs to be treated and hence removed. In the diagnostic culture, nothing is to be learned from a period of anxiety – the symptoms of anxiety are merely to be eliminated.

But the revolution Horwitz points at also hints at another pivotal development that the *DSM-III* instigated – namely the beginning of the proliferation of anxiety. Since the 1980s, there is strong evidence that the number of people diagnosed with anxiety and public reports of anxiety have gone up. Epidemiological studies indicate that vast numbers of people in western societies are suffering from anxiety (Horwitz 2013: 143). This tendency is backed by the birth cohort analysis made by Jean M. Twenge, which shows that the levels of anxiety and anxiety diagnosis reported in the USA between 1952 and 1992 have gone up significantly (Twenge 2000). More recently, a large Danish survey has shown that anxiety – especially among teenagers and adolescents – is the fastest-growing and most widely proliferated disorder in contemporary Danish society (Flachs *et al.* 2015). Hence, it seems quite pertinent to call our epoch the age of anxiety. It is my claim, however, that we cannot understand this development only by examining the internal transition of psychiatric thinking. The growing numbers of people diagnosed with anxiety are not just caused by alterations within psychiatric thinking. It is not just because the *DSM* changed its philosophy and shifted focus from aetiology to symptomatology that we are witnessing a bourgeoning rate of people with anxiety. In that respect I disagree with the argument of Allan Horwitz, who has stated that:

> it does not seem plausible that the upsurge in measured rates of anxiety represents a genuine epidemic of anxiety disorders. Instead, the putative growth of anxiety disorders since the implementation of the *DSM-III* seems to stem primarily from the use of diagnostic criteria that fail to actually distinguish natural from disordered anxiety.
>
> Horwitz 2013: 144

There is no doubt about the fact that the successful implementation of new diagnostic criteria of anxiety has paved some of the way for its proliferation. My point is, however, that this cannot account for the whole story. What we also need is an analysis of the socio-structural transformations that have supported the diagnostic understanding of anxiety and hence for its proliferation. Only by engaging ourselves in this are we able to understand why anxiety, in the contemporary age of anxiety, is perceived as an individualized disorder of societal significance. More specifically, we need an analysis of what it is in contemporary anxiety that informs us about current perceptions of order and pathology.

Anxieties in the age of anxiety

So far we have not defined what anxiety is – and that is no easy task. Anxiety is, indeed, a very complex phenomenon and it is beyond the scope of this chapter to go into depth with the many layers of anxiety. What is possible, however, is to give a broad definition of what anxiety entails and then move on to addressing the forms of anxiety that haunt contemporary society.

The condition of anxiety, most researchers would agree, is 'comprised of a complex emotional process which involves not only our thoughts, but also our physiology and behaviour' (Wilkinson 2001: 15). That is, anxiety consists of affective experiences, behavioural responses and bodily reactions. But, as already mentioned, the main arbiters of anxiety definitions in contemporary society are the diagnostic manuals – the *DSM-5* or the International Classification of Diseases *(ICD)-10*. It is in the realm of their medical logic to define anxiety as a syndrome that occurs independently of 'any unique qualities of the patients who carry its symptoms or of the period of human history when it appeared' (Horwitz 2013: 2). Pathological anxiety, then, consists first and foremost of the number and the severity of symptoms that people have in a given period of time. That logic is transferred unto a wide variety of different anxiety categories such as panic disorder (with or without agoraphobia); social phobias; obsessive-compulsive disorder; post-traumatic stress disorder; acute stress disorder; generalized anxiety disorders; and many others. These disorders are categorized as being distinct from one another and also from other mental disorders such as depression[6] and somatoform disorders. What is more, the definitions in these manuals make sharp distinctions between those people who have these disorders and those who don't. Again, the pool of symptoms and their severity connected with each of these disorders are decisive of those who are included into the category and those who are not.

If we take a closer look at some of the mentioned categories of anxiety, we are able to approach the overall argument of this chapter, namely that these disorders inform us about specific human traits that are socially constituted as pathological in contemporary society. More specifically, three of the most actualized types of anxiety are singled out: social phobia, panic disorder (without agoraphobia) and generalized anxiety disorder. These disorders are defined in the following manner in the *ICD-10*:

> **Generalized anxiety disorder**: Anxiety that is generalized and persistent but not restricted to, or even strongly predominating in, any particular environmental circumstances (i.e. it is 'free-floating'). The dominant symptoms are variable but include complaints of persistent nervousness, trembling, muscular tensions, sweating, light-headedness, palpitations, dizziness, and epigastric discomfort. Fears that the patient or a relative will shortly become ill or have an accident are often expressed.

Social phobias: Fear of scrutiny by other people leading to avoidance of social situations. More pervasive social phobias are usually associated with low self-esteem and fear of criticism. They may present as a complaint of blushing, hand tremor, nausea, or urgency of micturition, the patient sometimes being convinced that one of these secondary manifestations of their anxiety is the primary problem. Symptoms may progress to panic attacks.

Panic disorder: The essential feature is recurrent attacks of severe anxiety (panic), which are not restricted to any particular situation or set of circumstances and are therefore unpredictable. As with other anxiety disorders, the dominant symptoms include sudden onset of palpitations, chest pain, choking sensations, dizziness, and feelings of unreality (depersonalization or derealization). There is often also a secondary fear of dying, losing control, or going mad.

In order to legitimize why these disorders are singled out it seems adequate to refer to the fact that these are among the most proliferated anxiety disorders in contemporary western societies (Scott 2006; Fricchione 2004). Thus, it is more than likely that a vast number of people – including the readers of this book – can relate themselves to one of these disorders and their symptoms. If we take a closer look at the above-mentioned definitions, this is not particularly odd. By a first glance these definitions are quite broad, entailing a considerable number of human behaviours and emotions that are being scrutinized as problematic and signs of mental illness. In this sense it is not difficult to understand why scholars such as Horwitz refer to processes of pathologization when explaining the proliferation of these disorders (Horwitz 2013: 158). By pathologization, it is understood that diagnostic manuals such as the *ICD* and the *DSM* are failing to distinguish between natural and disordered anxiety, thereby promoting specific symptoms as pathological and hence instigating a breakdown of our conventional distinctions between problems in living and psychiatric disorders (see also Lau 2012). This perspective posits that the ongoing cultural process of pathologization implies that many traits and behaviours that used to be considered as normal human problems (sorrow, guilt, shyness, disruptive behaviour etc.) are now conceptualized as mental disorders that can be diagnosed and treated medically and therapeutically.[7] Perhaps the transformation of shyness into social phobia is the best indication of this process of pathologization, at least when it comes to issues of anxiety. As Christopher Lane (Lane 2007) and Susie Scott (Scott 2006) have shown, shyness has become an unhealthy state of mind in contemporary society and thereby transformed into a diagnosable mental illness in the form of social phobia. What was hitherto considered 'just shyness' has hence found its way into the specific diagnosis of social phobia, something that is largely enabled by the prevailing psychiatric mind-set of the diagnostic manuals, both Lane and Scott argue. The consequence is, according to the authors, that instead of providing clear-cut boundaries between natural and abnormal anxiety, the medical model of the diagnostic manuals in fact gives much leeway in pathologizing what was previously considered to be normal behaviour. What is more, this has paved the way for an increasing medicalization of shyness, as particularly Scott argues, and is thereby to be viewed as a central aspect of an overall development of medicalization of – and hence managing – social deviance per se that we are witnessing in late modern society (Scott 2006: 148).

The pathologization of these kinds of anxiety is, no doubt about it, partly responsible for their widespread proliferation. But again, this explanation cannot account for the entire development. The process of pathologization per se, does not explain why these particular mental disorders are socially constituted as pathological. Or, to be more precise, it does not explain why these particular symptoms are understood as signifiers of mental illness in contemporary society. In this respect it is pivotal to be aware of the fact that mental disorders, when inscribed in the diagnostic manuals, are constituted by symptoms. Unlike somatic illnesses, in which symptoms are signs of a particular disease – blood in the stools is indicative of colon cancer (but is not necessarily cancer per se) – the symptoms of mental illnesses *are* the disease. The variety, length and severity of the symptoms account for the disease that can be diagnosed. So in this respect it seems quite important to base the analyses of our particular age of anxiety on the symptoms that constitute the aforementioned kinds of anxiety. When invoking such a gaze on the definitions of general anxiety disorder, social phobia and panic disorder one rather obvious element of the symptoms arises. They evolve around individual loss of control of one's life, particularly concerning the individual mind (sense of self) and the body. This loss manifests itself in different ways in the different forms of anxiety, ranging from feelings of depersonalization, low self-esteem and nervousness to lightheadedness, blushing and dizziness. This loss of control is not restricted to any particular situations, albeit social phobias and panic disorder are more likely to occur in social situations in which the individual is to take part.

Of course, a loss of control is also a pertinent part of other mental disorders – for example, depression. In depression, the gradual experience of losing control over one's life is often followed by feelings of helplessness and a sense of hopelessness, true hallmarks of depression (Ratcliffe 2015). American psychiatrist Dan G. Blazer even goes as far as to state that 'The swelling prevalence of depression in Western society perhaps reflects and increasingly dominant hopelessness within society' (Blazer 2005: 154). In Blazer's account, the connection between the ascent of depression and the loss of hope can be analysed in detail by extracting eight themes associated with the loss of hope. These are: loss of story; loss of language; loss of self; loss of unity; loss of trust; loss of orientation; loss of meaning; and, finally, nihilism (ibid.: 154–8). Without going into detail with these eight themes, I would like to raise two questions concerning Blazer's thesis. First: is contemporary western society really experiencing a general loss of hope? I would answer in the negative. I would rather argue – as I will do in the next paragraph – that we are witnessing a significant change in the social norms and rules that is altering the societal conditions for the emergence of social pathologies such as depression and anxiety disorders. Second: can we rank the loss of hope put forward by Blazer alongside the loss of control that I argue is the common feature of the anxieties in question? Again, I would argue no. The difference is that Blazer claims the bourgeoning rates of depression are caused by the overall loss of hope while I claim that the above-mentioned anxieties – and hence the loss of control connected with them – are constituted by and are a reaction to new societal conditions of what it means to be a human being in contemporary society. The main point is that these forms of anxiety are reflecting types of individual loss of control – feelings and behaviours – that are socially unwelcome in the cultural climate of contemporary late modern society. But, at the same time, the cultural climate in contemporary society, I will argue, is fostering the societal conditions that support the emergence of these types of anxiety. The question is, in which way?

Anxieties as signs of social pathology in contemporary society

The concept of social pathology has, ever since it was proliferated and popularized by Émile Durkheim, been controversial. The mere idea that society can be sick, and that society can cause harm to individual organisms and psyches, is not straightforward and critique has been raised. In his relatively critical article about the notion of social pathology, French sociologist Alain Ehrenberg writes the following:

> The idea underlying the adjunction of the adjective 'social' to the substantive 'pathology' is that mental pathologies are the product of our social relationships, that they reveal something about our mores and lifestyles, and that there is a moral, social and political lesson to be drawn from this type of pathology.
>
> Ehrenberg 2013: 11

Although Ehrenberg does not discard this idea entirely, he does not embrace it either. In fact, he is critical about the idea of society producing the conditions through which mental pathologies are created. As he has written in some of his previous work: 'we are witnessing a change of the social status of psychic suffering – and not a *psychological aggravation* of the condition of individuals in "depressive society"' (Ehrenberg 2010a: 9). In fact, Ehrenberg is arguing that the altered social status of psychic suffering – here understood as increased awareness and public attention – has paved the way for the bourgeoning rates of mental illnesses that we are confronted with in contemporary society.

In a similar vein, German social philosopher Axel Honneth is also challenging the scope of the concept of social pathology (Honneth 2014). He does so by investigating the concept via the thoughts of German social-psychologist

Alexander Mitscherlich and Sigmund Freud. In Honneth's perspective both of these theorists are two narrow in their analytical scope. He writes:

> At first, Mitscherlich ties the existence of a social disease to the existence of a conspicuous number of the members of society suffering from symptoms of a psychic abnormality to such a degree that they consult in droves physicians or therapists. Without this first indicator of a suffering from psychic functional impairment, experienced en masse, there seems to be no reason, in Mitscherlich's picture, to look for deeper disturbances in the process of social integration. Similarly, for Freud, whose cultural diagnoses clearly set the example for Mitscherlich's inquiry, the neurologists first need to register a rapid increase in a specific class of only psychologically explainable illnesses before the sociologically invested analyst can go on to search for their causes in the societal apparatus.
>
> Ibid.: 686

At a certain level, there is nothing wrong with these observations, Honneth argues. The problem arises, however, if one establishes a too intimate bond between conspicuous societal tendencies and the increase in symptoms that are manifested in widespread illness among individuals. And Honneth thinks both Freud and Mitscherlich fall prey to this mistake. If the analysis of social pathologies rests almost entirely on this premise, the argumentation is going to be too vague – even flawed, Honneth claims. In order to speak of social pathologies, or of diseases of social life, Honneth believes a transition to the 'independent organizational unit of society, which is irreducible to the sum of its individual members' behavior' (ibid.: 689), is required. Thus, we need to broaden our analytical scope substantially and utilize the concept of social pathologies accordingly. However, as mentioned, Honneth is not claiming that the rise in mental pathologies or psychic suffering is indifferent in the analysis of social pathologies. As he writes: 'There would be no reason to give thought to potential "diseases" of society if the failures of individual socialization did not generally reflect themselves in behavioral abnormalities of the members of society' (ibid.: 690). Thus, it is all about the scope of things and hence about the usage of the concept of social pathologies.

In my perspective, both Ehrenberg and Honneth are directing attention to important issues. But I also disagree with them. In relation to Ehrenberg, I simply think he is off the mark in only considering the changed social status of psychic suffering when accounting for increased rates of mental illnesses. I mean, there is hardly any doubt about the fact that psychic suffering has a totally different social status now compared to 40 years ago. Hence, there is an increasing societal awareness about psychic suffering as well as an extended perception of what psychic suffering really is. I have already mentioned the process of pathologization as one pivotal aspect of this development. But, there is also a societal development that one has to take into consideration when accounting for the bourgeoning rates of, for example, different kinds of anxiety, I will argue. In relation to Honneth, I almost entirely concur with his reasoning. One cannot reduce the analysis of social pathologies to increasing levels of mental illnesses. Social pathologies might very well manifest themselves in other – and more collective – ways than in individual psychic malaises. This does not entail, as Honneth is well aware, that we should neglect the analysis of increased levels of individual psychic suffering as signs of social pathologies. In fact, I would argue, the need to make these analyses is a matter of utmost importance, especially in the light of contemporary society trying to reduce particular psychic malaises to individual problems. That is, there is a widespread tendency in contemporary society to individualize problems that could, in fact, be seen as structurally stimulated.

It is in line with this reasoning that I argue the following. In our historical epoch the above-mentioned types of anxiety are not only manifesting themselves as the seamy side of a societally recognized normality, the bourgeoning rates of these anxieties are also present because of increasing societal pressure to perform ceaselessly. What is normality, then, in our late modern society? American sociologists Luigi Esposito and Fernando Perez have answered this question by putting late modern society and contemporary neoliberal society on the same footing. They write:

> subjects in a neoliberal society are considered normal and functional only when they show a willingness to compete with others for the things they need or desire and when they assume 'personal responsibility' for their own problems. In contrast, any person who fails to display these qualities is assumed to fail not only as an economic actor but also as a responsible being. In fact, failing to display these sorts of behavioural and/or attitudinal qualities is very commonly attributed to some type of personal dysfunction or pathology.
>
> Esposito and Perez 2014: 421

The claim is quite straightforward. Being normal – and hence functional – is only possible if one internalizes the inclination to compete with others and by assuming personal responsibility for all aspects of one's own life. The functional aspect of being normal is quite narrowly understood. Functional equals being able to perform adequately on the ever-changing labour market, hence being able to address the required competences and normative demands. Only the functional are able to compete with others, which is why the internalization of the necessary competences and normative demands are crucial. So, which are the required competences and normative demands? We know that a clear-cut definition of the required competences is impossible. It is hard to predict the future. Therefore, vague categorizations are used. These are, more often than not, connected with – and understood as the same thing as – the normative demands put forward in our historical epoch. In order to understand these we can turn to French sociologists Luc Boltanski and Eve Chiapello.

In their seminal study on the emergence of the new spirit of capitalism, they have coined a comprehensive list of normative demands individuals in contemporary society are confronted with in order to be attractive for the labour market. These, all collected under the heading of endless activity, are: flexibility, polyvalence, adaptability, mobility, connect-ability, versatility and the ability to be open, friendly, funny, self-aware and easy-going. All of these qualities – in fact put forward as demands – are markers of a persons' employability – what Boltanski and Chiapello refer to as 'markers of great men' (Boltanski and Chiapello 2005: 114). Thus, great – employable – men [and women] are able to internalize these qualities and employ them in competition with others in regard to who is the most attractive person for a particular position. Small men [and women] – or what they refer to as 'little persons' – on the contrary, are incapable of being flexible, versatile etc., which ultimately grounds them as unemployable and hence without the necessary means of entering competitive relationships (ibid.: 119). Thus, if we follow the claim of Esposito and Perez, the little persons in Boltanski and Chiapello's terminology are attributed to being dysfunctional or even pathological. If we look at the definitions of the above-mentioned types of anxiety, the analysis is – I believe – quite easily legitimized. The markers of great men are totally absent in the definitions of the types of anxiety. Instead of flexibility and adaptability, fear and nervousness are the hallmarks of anxiety. Instead of being an easy-going and self-aware, low self-esteem and depersonalization characterize these anxieties, and so on. No one who is struggling with these symptoms is capable of internalizing the normative demands required to be a great person. In that respect, the absence of taking responsibility of one's life – and thus not being able to compete with others on the grounds of these normative demands – is considered to be the exact opposite of normality and therefore pathological.

I would also argue, however, that the demand in itself to live in accordance with these normative demands – and hence the ongoing attempt to internalize them – can lead to the above-mentioned anxieties. What is crucial in this understanding is the fact that the normative demands have been institutionalized. In this respect one could talk about the role of the media – the Facebook generation etc. where the demands to constantly compete and show that one leads a good, healthy and interesting life is affecting people 24/7. This is combined with the fact that, in contemporary institutional settings – such as kindergartens, schools and universities – the pupils and students are constantly confronted with curricula that support the overall idea of internalizing these normative demands (Pedersen 2011). That is, they are confronted with the idealizations of these demands and hence with the overall positive outcome of their display. In that respect, they are also confronted with the negative outcome of a lack of their successful internalization. The constant awareness of this – and the mere confrontation with these powerful demands – is, in fact, putting immense pressure on individuals to perform accordingly. This pressure is actually augmented by the fact that these demands – however difficult they might be to internalize – are wrapped in positive connotations. Because who would not like to act responsibly in respect to one's own life? Who would not like to be considered a great person? Who would not like to be flexible, adaptable, funny, etc.? We all would – but the fact of the matter is that more and more people are showing signs of the exact opposite. And, especially concerning the types of anxiety in question here, more and more young people and adolescents are struck down with this 'disorder'. One of the reasons why that is, I would claim, is exactly because of the fact that they are institutionally confronted with the demands. Young people today are increasingly reacting negatively to what I refer to as the chronic stressor of adhering to these normative demands. According to Canadian sociologist Blair Wheaton, chronic stressors are defined as ongoing pressure on a person's mental well-being caused by difficulties of coping adequately with this pressure (Wheaton 1999). In this respect I would argue that one central explanation of why more young people are showing signs of and given the diagnosis of anxiety is due to the fact that the pressure – the chronic stressor – to internalize these normative demands is causing the opposite. They lose control instead of gaining control over these normative demands. So, instead of leading to flexible, adaptable young people who are able to compete with each other and ultimately become employable, an increasing amount of young people are facing anxieties.

Instead of dealing with the social aspects of these pathologies, the common reaction against this development is individualized treatment. That is, various forms of psychopharmacology and cognitive behavioural therapy are the most prescribed forms of treatment for these anxieties. The overall logic of these types of treatment is the individual removal of the symptoms connected with the pathological behaviour. The symptoms are distressing and should hence be eliminated. That is, the focus of the treatment is elimination of symptoms in order for the individual to return to a life free of symptoms. In that respect the treatments are adhering to the ideal of individual responsibility for one's problems in life without taking any particular social aspects of the symptoms into consideration. The anxieties in question are simply malaises that no individual should endure – therefore they should be eradicated.

The future of anxiety

In her psychoanalytically informed analysis of anxiety in contemporary society, Renata Salecl not only delivers a cultural critique of what, in her mind, paves the way for increasing anxiety. She also warns us about the dangers of perceiving anxiety as something we should do our utmost to eliminate. Anxiety – understood in the right way – is not only, she contends, a negative emotion but also a fruitful phenomenon we should learn from. She ends her book by writing: 'Society without anxiety would similarly be a dangerous place to live in' (Salecl 2004: 148). In what way dangerous, we might ask?

I would argue that are two ways of answering this question. The first answer is quite straightforward. Anxiety is, or at least could be, a compelling yardstick for measuring socio-political developments. That is, if we do not have anxiety as a kind of a backstop for political and social incentives and policies, we are lacking a very powerful stop-sign. In that respect one could actually argue that we need even more anxiety today, considering the current political and socio-cultural developmental tendencies. The second, I believe, is more interesting in relation to this chapter. This answer concerns the ways in which the presence of anxiety is orienting and informing us about the quasi-anthropological human need for boundaries. In fact, the above-mentioned analysis of what it entails to be a human being – or a subject – in contemporary society, is very much a story about blurring boundaries. It is not a question of missing boundaries, but instead of social rules and norms that are dependent on extremely elastic boundaries. My contention is that the social rules and norms that I have been discussing are so powerful and compelling because they scrutinize – and in a certain sense constantly erase – limitations. In contemporary society there should be no limits as to what you can do – as long as you follow the prerequisites of the social norms and rules, that is. Hence, there is a socio-cultural inclination not to let yourself get bothered or constrained by limitations – indeed, an institutional demand not to be caught in the straightjacket of socially or culturally imposed confines. Especially for young people, when it comes to questions of education and future job-realizations, the demand to constantly explore the ever-changing potentialities is present. It is only by doing so that they are able to flourish and realize themselves in a satisfying manner. Ultimately, then, I will argue, the mere idea of blurry boundaries is so powerful because it is heralded as individual freedom. Richard Sennett has, when talking about the cultural norm of adaptability, addressed this aspect. He writes: 'we imagine being open to change, being adaptable, as qualities of character needed for free action – the human being free because capable of change' (Sennett 1998: 48).

In such a socio-cultural constellation there is, of course, no room for anxiety. Anxiety is, for lack of better words, a party-pooper to the contemporary understanding of free – and hence normal – individual adaptation to the presiding social norms and rules. Therein lies the danger, I would claim. The danger of upholding the idea that anxiety is only to be perceived as a restriction to individual freedom and not as a marker of the necessary limitation to this freedom.

So, is there such a thing as a future for anxiety? I would argue that there are severe dangers involved in neglecting anxiety and only envisaging it as something we should eradicate. Perhaps we should pause and learn from the massive proliferation of anxieties in contemporary society instead of just trying to reject its pedagogical values by addressing them as individual malaises and hence not social pathologies. Perhaps!

Notes

1 The other two main tasks are: theoretical construction of concepts and empirical testing of theoretical assumptions.

2 I do not wish to pretend that all sociologists agree that the discipline should engage itself in diagnoses of the times. English sociologist Mike Savage has written an article entitled 'Against epochalism' that argues for the serious pitfalls of this endeavour (Savage 2009).

3 In a later article, 'How an age of anxiety became an age of depression', Allan V. Horwitz has elaborated on this argument (Horwitz 2010).

4 In the next chapter this line of argumentation will be analysed and debated.
5 In his study *Suicide*, Émile Durkheim mentions neurasthenia several times and comments on its societal proliferation (Durkheim 2006).
6 We are well aware of the fact that depression is the most common coexisting disorder in patients with most types of anxiety disorder. This is not, however, the same as saying that these disorders are similar. In the diagnostic manuals they are sharply separated.
7 One pivotal aspect of the diagnostic culture is precisely the emergence of multiple diagnoses that encapsulates an increasing selection of human behaviour as signs of mental pathology. Among the more curious diagnoses that have entered the *DSM-5* is hoarding disorder, nicotine dependency disorder and premenstrual dysphoric disorder (PMDD). Now, these conditions might be problematic but are they really mental disorders? Or have they become pathologized due to a lack of thorough distinction between the normal and the pathological?

References

Auden, W.H. (1948): *The Age of Anxiety*. London: Faber & Faber.

Bauman, Z. (2000): *Liquid Modernity*. Cambridge: Polity Press.

Beck, U. and Bonss, W. (eds) (2001): *Die Modernisierung der Moderne*. Frankfurt am Main: Suhrkamp.

Boltanski, L. and Chiapello, È. (2005): *The New Spirit of Capitalism*. London: Verso.

Beard, G (1869): Neurasthenia, or nervous exhaustion. *The Boston Medical and Surgical Journal*: 217–21.

Blazer, D.G. (2005): *The Age of Melancholy: 'Major Depression' and its Discontents*. London: Routledge.

Brinkmann, S. and Petersen, A. (eds) (2015): *Diagnoser – perspektiver, kritik og diskussion*. Aarhus: Klim.

Callan, E. (1965): Allegory in Auden's The Age of Anxiety. *Twentieth Century Literature*, 10: 155 65.

Durkheim, E. (2006): *On Suicide*. London: Penguin.

Ehrenberg, A. (2010a): Society of discontent or discontent in society? http://www.booksandideas.net/Society-of-Discontent-or.html (accessed 25 June 2016).

Ehrenberg, A. (2010b): *The Weariness of the Self: Diagnosing the History of Depression in the Contemporary Age*. Montreal and Kingston: McGill-Queen's University Press.

Ehrenberg, A. (2013): The notion of social pathology: a case study of Narcissus in American society. In: Keohane, K. and Petersen, A. (eds), *The Social Pathologies of Contemporary Civilization*. Farnham: Ashgate.

Esposito, L. and Perez, F.M. (2014): Neoliberalism and the commodification of mental health. *Humanity and Society*, 38(4): 414–42.

Flachs, E.M., Eriksen, L., Koch, M.B., Ryd, J.T., Dibba, E., Skov-Ettrup, L. and Juel, K. (2015): *Sygdomsbyrden i Danmark – Sygdomme*. København: Sundhedsstyrelsen.

Freud, S. (1959/1926): *Inhibitions, Symptoms and Anxiety*. New York: W.W. Norton.

Fricchione, G. (2004): Generalized anxiety disorder. *The New England Journal of Medicine*, 351: 675–82.

Giddens, A. (1991): *Modernity and Self-Identity: Self and Society in the Late Modern Age*. Cambridge: Polity Press.

Honneth, A. (2014): The diseases of society. approaching a nearly impossible concept. Social *Research: An International Quarterly*, 81(3): 683–703.

Horwitz, A.V. (2002): *Creating Mental Illness*. Chicago: Chicago University Press.

Horwitz, A.V. (2010): How an age of anxiety became an age of depression. *Milbank Quarterly* 88: 112–38.

Horwitz, A.V. (2013): *Anxiety. A Short History*. Baltimore, MD: Johns Hopkins University Press.

Horwitz, A.V. and Wakefield, J.C. (2005): The age of depression. *The Public Interest*, 158: 39–58.

Kierkegaard, S. (1980): *On the Concept of Anxiety*. Princeton, NJ: Princeton University Press.

Lane, C. (2007). *Shyness: How Normal Behavior Became a Sickness*. New Haven, CT: Yale University Press.

Lau, R.W.K. (2012): Understanding contemporary modernity through the trends of therapy and life-'skills' training. *Current Sociology*, 60(1): 81–100.

Lichtblau, K. (1995): Sociology and the diagnosis of the times, or: the reflexivity of modernity. *Theory, Culture and Society*, 12: 25–52.

Lipovetsky, G. (2005): *Hypermodern Times*. Cambridge: Polity Press.

Lyotard, J.-F. (1981): *La condition postmoderne: Rapport sur le savoir*. Paris: Éditions de Minuit.

Parish, J. (2001): The age of anxiety. *The Editorial Board of the Sociological Review*: 1–16.

Pedersen, O.K. (2011): *Konkurrencestaten*. København: Hans Reitzels Forlag.

Ratcliffe, M. (2015): *Experiences of Depression: A Study in Phenomenology*. Oxford: Oxford University Press.

Rosenberg, C.E. (2002): The tyranny of diagnosis: specific entities and individual experience. *Milbank Quarterly*, 2: 237–60.

Salecl, R. (2004): *On Anxiety*. London: Routledge.

Savage, M. (2009): Against epochalism: an analysis of conceptions of change in British sociology. *Cultural Sociology*, 3(2): 217–38.

Scott, S. (2006): The medicalisation of shyness: from social misfits to social fitness. *Sociology of Health and Illness*, 28: 133–53.

Sennett, R. (1998): *The Corrosion of Character: The Personal Consequences of Work in the New Capitalism*. New York: Norton.

Shorter, E. (1997): *A History of Psychiatry: From the Era of the Asylum to the Age of Prozac*. New York: John Wiley and Sons.

Shorter, E. (2013): *How Everyone Became Depressed*. Oxford: Oxford University Press.

Twenge, J.M. (2000): The age of anxiety? Birth cohort change in anxiety and neuroticism, 1952–1993. *Journal of Personality and Social Psychology*, 79(6): 1007–21.

Wheaton, B. (1999): The nature of stressors. In: Horwitz, A.V. and Scheid, T.L. (eds), *A Handbook for the Study of Mental Health: Social Contexts, Theories, and Systems*. Cambridge: Cambridge University Press.

World Health Organization: *ICD-10*. In: http://apps.who.int/classifications/icd10/browse/2015/en#/F41.0 (accessed 25 June 2016).

Wilkinson, I. (2001): *Anxiety in a Risk Society*. London: Routledge.

4 Sadean depression and the work of culture

Bert van den Bergh

Introduction: nobody saw it coming

Recently, within a brief space of time, two startling incidents were reported in the Dutch media. The first was the suicide of Joost Zwagerman, an author celebrated because of his novels and poetry, but also due to his continuous passionate written and oral defence of the power of art, especially as a regular guest in the popular TV talkshow *De wereld draait door.*[1] Besides that, Zwagerman published in the last part of his writing career several essays on the themes of depression and suicide. The context of this was highly personal: his father had made an unsuccessful suicide attempt and one of his best friends, also a writer, had struggled throughout his life with severe depression and suicidal thoughts, until in the end he was formally allowed to carry out euthanasia because of 'unendurable mental and physical suffering'. To the very last day Zwagerman set his face against the death wish of his friend, in line with the denunciation put forward in his writings of what he called 'the done-with-life school'. Shortly before his death he emphasized once again in an interview that, although depression was familiar territory for himself as well, suicide had always remained 'a no-go area'. Nevertheless he finally went there.

A few days after Zwagerman's death his friend Bram Bakker, psychiatrist and writer, published an article in one of the leading Dutch newspapers with the title 'Nobody knows what came over Joost' (NRC 12 September 2015). We shouldn't ask why he did it, Bakker states there, because what he did is incomprehensible. What we need to do, the psychiatrist continues, is 'come up with something that makes depression more widely known' because talking about this 'terrible disease' is still too painful and too shameful. At the end of his article Bakker therefore announces a Depression Gala, which would take place on the next Blue Monday,[2] first, to commemorate Joost Zwagerman and others 'who lost the battle against depression' and, second, 'to further emancipate psychiatry'. Four months later, on 26 January 2016, the gala indeed was held in a suburban theatre in Amsterdam. The double aim of the evening was to help stop this disorder from being taboo and to raise funds for specific depression initiatives. Legitimizing the paradoxical format of an entertaining evening on a mental disorder, depression was put on a par with 'other diseases' like cancer and amyotrophic lateral sclerosis (ALS), for which similar events are organized regularly. A number of celebrities performed a sort of depression coming-out, Joost Zwagerman was commemorated several times and the Dutch Minister of Health, Welfare and Sports gave a speech in which she promised several million euro for the fight against this society-disrupting disease.[3]

The second shocking occurrence reported in the autumn of 2015 was a string of suicides in the Dutch 'Bible Belt' village of Wezep, where, in a space of one year, five young people – one girl and four boys – took their own lives. An article in the same newspaper that published Bakker's text, appearing only three weeks later, recounted how the mayor of the municipality of Wezep called a halt to the silence surrounding the village suicides. The days our community could look away are gone, stated the mayor. 'What does it take to be there for each other?' he asked (NRC 5 October 2015). The community needs to act boldly now: 'a policy document is not going to improve this; all Wezep has to be mobilized, has to take responsibility'. A 'taskforce' was set up in Wezep, consisting of mothers of those who had committed suicide, some other engaged village inhabitants, a vicar and a social worker. The idea was to provide 'vitamin A', as the mayor called it, meaning the 'a' of attention. That is, indeed, what children need, the mother of one of the suicide victims is quoted in the article: 'we have to put away our phones at the end of the day and ask each other how the day was, we need to make things discussible'. Also in this second article the word 'taboo' is used.

The title given to the Wezep story has a similar ring to that of the article on Zwagerman: 'Nobody in Wezep has noticed how down Jim was'. Jim is the name of the last youngster who ended his life. Nobody noticed, nobody knew, nobody could know. The harrowing similarity between these two stories is that the suicide came out of the blue, the striking difference is 'culture of speech' versus 'culture of silence'. For the intellectual inner circle of Zwagerman almost everything was 'discussible', whereas the Protestant villagers of Wezep were silent about many things. It does not seem to have made a difference. In both contexts the cases of extreme depression were cases of extreme isolation. No one in the inner circle of Zwagerman and no one in the close community Wezep considers itself to be in the end knew what was going on. These depressed persons had become unreachable, they were in a state of utter isolation, like expressed in the motto Zwagerman chose for his suicide essay collection *Door eigen hand. Zelfmoord en de nabestaanden*,[4] a quote from Al Alvarez's *The Savage God*: 'Once a man decides to take his own life he enters a shut-off, impregnable but wholly convincing world where every detail fits and each incident reinforces his decision' (Alvarez 2002/1971: 145).

Depression alarm

A completely closed world, a state of extreme isolation is also at the heart of many autobiographical accounts of depression. It is the 'immense and aching solitude' of William Styron, for instance, or 'the most isolated place on earth' of Sally Brampton[5] (Ratcliffe 2015: 102). 'So many people have asked me what to do for depressed friends and relatives,' Andrew Solomon writes in his acclaimed *The Noonday Demon: An Anatomy of Depression*, 'and my answer is actually simple: blunt their isolation' (Solomon 2002: 436f).[6] These blunting attempts had failed in the cases of Zwagerman and the Wezep youngsters. Because of a taboo, so the widely shared explanation goes. Ultimate hopelessness of the suicidal is succeeded by embarrassed helplessness of the survivors. Which then is parried by a call to mobilize the community, break the taboo, pay closer attention. One sounds the alarm for a hidden evil, an insidious disease: the intangible Black Dog.[7]

Yet the depression alarm has been sounding on all sides already for quite some time[8] – sounded, for instance, by the European Depression Association (EDA), an alliance of organizations, researchers, health care professionals and patients from 19 European countries. In its *Depression Manifesto* it states that depression is 'a common, serious and in some cases, life-threatening condition, affecting around 30 million people in Europe' and thereby 'one of the greatest public health challenges in Europe'. As such, the EDA appeals to governments 'for immediate and decisive policy action to ensure that depression is prioritised within actions to improve health in general and mental health in particular' (EDA n.d.: 2) Each year, on 1 October, the EDA organizes a European Depression Day in Brussels, during which policy makers and members of the European Parliament discuss possible policies and legislation relating to this major socio-economic problem. Throughout October various events are held across Europe to raise awareness of depression. This is needed, the EDA states, since:

> despite the prevalence and burden of depression and the fact that there are effective interventions for it that cover the full range of symptoms, fewer than half of those affected in the world (in some countries, fewer than 10%) receive such care.
>
> Ibid.: 3

War is declared on a common enemy: 'Together we will fight depression, together we will win' (ibid.: 11).

The statistics mentioned by the EDA are borrowed from the WHO, the United Nations watchdog that presently is sounding the depression alarm on a global scale, estimating that 350 million people of all ages suffer from this disorder. The WHO claims that depression is 'the leading cause of disability world-wide' and 'a major contributor to the overall global burden of disease'. This claim is presented in terms of 'global crisis', 'public health priority' and 'hidden burden'. Like the EDA, the WHO states that, although already since the 1990s there is rumour of a depression epidemic, the factual burden of this mental disorder is still heavily underrated: 'Yet, many of us are in denial. Depression remains hidden – not treated or talked about.' And consequently the WHO summons us to take action: 'Let's recognize and deal with it.'[9]

But what exactly is it that we are dealing with? We are threatened, so the prevailing thought is, by a disease which to a large extent still works in the dark. Depression is said to be 'taboo' and a 'hidden burden'.[10] So we need to expose the spectre and try to neutralize it, and we should try much harder than we already do because, though depression is already recognized as a 'common disease', the disease is much more common than we think, according to the EDA, the WHO and many other health care stakeholders. But what 'disease' is it that we have to contend with? According to the leading text of the global antidepression enterprise, the *DSM*, the core of the disorder in question is either an enduring sadness or a lasting loss of interest or pleasure: 'The essential feature of a major depressive episode is a period of at least 2 weeks during which there is either depressed mood or the loss of interest or pleasure in nearly all activities' (APA 2013: 163). So there should be anhedonia or dejection, but not necessarily so: 'In children and adolescents, the mood may be irritable rather than sad' (ibid.). And there needs to be more:

> The individual must also experience at least four additional symptoms drawn from a list that includes changes in appetite or weight, sleep, and psychomotor activity; decreased energy; feelings of worthlessness or guilt; difficulty thinking, concentrating, or making decisions; or recurrent thoughts of death or suicidal ideation or suicide plans or attempts. To count toward a major depressive episode, a symptom must either be newly present or must have clearly worsened compared with the person's pre-episode status. The symptoms must persist for most of the day, nearly every day, for at least 2 consecutive weeks.
>
> Ibid.

And finally, next to all of this, there need to be some accompanying factors: 'The episode must be accompanied by clinically significant distress or impairment in social, occupational, or other important areas of functioning' (ibid.).

Note that feelings of isolation are not classified as major symptoms – 'Criterion A' – but as *possible* accompaniments. I join with the British philosopher Matthew Ratcliffe, who in his recent *Experiences of Depression* marks this as a capital mistake: 'Impaired interpersonal relations are not an "effect" of depression experiences but absolutely central to them' (Ratcliffe 2015: 218). From a phenomenological perspective – which is the one Ratcliffe takes, along with other authors I will refer to in this chapter – it is not so much a feeling of sadness but an experience of isolation which is at the heart (or bottom) of 'depression'. The thesis I want to explore in this chapter is that of depression as a basic disconnectedness or distunement, which happens on a primordial, affective, pre-reflective, pre-intentional, pre-subjective level – that is, a level that precedes a separation of subject and object, individual and world. Furthermore, I will link this primordial distunement to the 'post-modern condition' of the contemporary subject, its 'isolist' or 'Sadean' position, as analysed by French philosopher Dany-Robert Dufour in his works on what he terms the 'liberal cultural revolution'. The 'anthropological mutation' Dufour speaks of, which is also explained in Chapter 2 of this volume, involves – and this is the second thesis of this chapter – a collective destructive confrontation with the 'isolist' or 'Sadean' position, a confrontation that manifests itself among other things as the so-called 'depression epidemic' which in recent decades has spread across the globe.

Neo-Kraepelinian revolution

Is depression perhaps a 'fashionable disease' – a disease that makes sense only within a specific historical context? Or, in other words and according to the definition in the *DSM*: should we take depression as a 'cultural syndrome'? For culture-specific types of disorders the *DSM* uses the latter term, which is defined as follows: 'clusters of symptoms and attributions that tend to co-occur among individuals in specific cultural groups, communities, or contexts and that are recognized locally as coherent patterns of experience' (APA 2013: 758).[11] These 'cultural syndromes' are opposed to *DSM* syndromes, although, at the same time, the *DSM* admits that the latter mostly came into being as the former: 'many *DSM* diagnoses can be understood as operationalized prototypes that started out as cultural syndromes, and became widely accepted as a result of their clinical and research utility' (ibid.). Do 'depressive disorders', then, belong to the 'many *DSM* diagnoses' that can be considered as, to put it like this, successful cultural syndromes? What would happen if we did this and thereby, one could say, kept to the letter of the *DSM*? Is depression our contemporary cultural syndrome, just like, for instance, neurasthenia was around the turn of the nineteenth to the twentieth century?[12] For a brief while, then, neurasthenia, or 'nervous exhaustion', was at the heart of our 'cultural idiom of distress', as the 'American nervousness' that came across the Atlantic towards Europe. The rapid rise of this phenomenon was succeeded by an equally quick decline.[13] Will the lot that fell to neurasthenia – suffering from modernity and 'modernization' – also fall to depression – suffering from late modernity and 'globalization'? Will this 'common disease' before long also wane and wither? There are no signs yet that this will be the case. The depression alarm is still in full swing. The WHO presents depression as 'the leading cause of disability worldwide'. The *DSM* and allied systems[14] have a strong grip on mental health care all over the world. Insurance companies demand that mental health care professionals act in accordance with it. Worldwide, people are forced to speak in terms that are heavily debated. What are we talking about when we talk about depression?

Actually we don't know, says the American psychiatrist and historian of psychiatry Edward Shorter. In *How Everyone Became Depressed: The Rise and Fall of the Nervous Breakdown* he distinguishes two kinds of depression: real depression or melancholia and depression-that-is-not-depression (Shorter 2013: 15, 80, 88, 127, 184). When we talk about depression, so Shorter claims, we, in fact, mostly talk about something else. What then? Shorter's suggestion is 'nerves', or more specifically, 'nervous illness' or 'nervous syndrome' (ibid.: ix). For Shorter it makes sense to return to a narrative from a century ago because that narrative considered the phenomenon that we now mistakenly call 'depression' as a disease of the entire body, instead of as 'mood disorder', so a disease of the mind only. Shorter not only intends to separate 'melancholia' from 'nonmelancholic mood disorder'[15] or 'depression', he also wants to get rid of the latter concept once and for all. Most of the people that are diagnosed as suffering from this mental disorder, so he claims, are not really ill. They are chiefly 'unhappy, aggrieved, tired, anxious, uncomfortable', or they have 'nothing at all really wrong' (ibid.: 171). Why then call this form of 'wretchedness' depression? Let us, for the time being, call them 'nervous', Shorter suggests. Let us return to a narrative in which the focus was on the following symptom complex: extreme fatigue, mild depression (so as a symptom only), mild anxiety, certain somatic symptoms (like chronic pain, insomnia and disordered bowel function) and some sort of obsessive thinking (ibid.: 11). Let us call this complex 'nervous syndrome'.[16]

On the last page of his book, Shorter presents a 'lesson' for patients:

> Millions of people have been led to believe that they are depressed when in fact their illness involves much more than their mood – it involves their entire brain and body. It is the whole that has to be treated, not the mood as such – because their feelings might well reflect demoralization, discouragement, discomfort, or disarray, but not depression.
>
> Ibid.: 198

What Shorter means by 'the whole' he already made clear in the introductory chapter of the book:

> In emphasizing nerves and the whole body rather than just mood, we join a worthy tradition of biological thinking in psychiatry, seeing so-called mental illness as brain disease, not the kind of frank pathological brain lesions studied by neurologists, but disorders of neural biology.
>
> Ibid.: 3f

And although he acknowledges that 'impulses from the brain are modified by thought, culture, and society before they turn into behavior', the focus is fixed on the 'deep story' of neurobiology. From a phenomenological angle, as will be discussed later in this chapter, the focus is on another 'deep story', which also involves the 'whole body', but 'body' then understood in a rather different way. And also 'mood' and 'affect' are conceived differently, one could say on a 'deeper' level – that is to say the 'internal' level of individual *experience* which at the same time is a *social* experience. This way, depression is linked to a primordial, intercorporeal, interaffective attunement of subject (or 'presubject') and world.

But first I would like to return to Shorter's argument because, concerning the concept of 'major depression', he certainly has a point. The symptomatographical[17] definition of this disorder in the *DSM* often does not seem to cover properly the personal accounts of the experiences of the so-called depressed.[18] Why is that? How did this concept come into being? By mistake, is Shorter's answer. He calls 'major depression' a 'disastrous concept' and a 'scientific travesty', and the introduction of it in *DSM-III* in 1980 a 'historic defeat' (Shorter 2013: 113, 171, 141). For psychoanalytically inspired psychiatry – which dominated the USA from the 1940s (Shorter 1997: 160ff) – specific diagnostic entities were of minor importance. Symptoms had to be taken as symbolic manifestations which needed to be interpreted adequately. The focus was on the total personality and the whole of personal life experience. One reasoned on the basis of a disease continuum and not of discrete disease categories. A strict separation between normality and pathology was rejected (Mayes and Horwitz 2005: 249f). Robert Spitzer – a psychoanalytically trained psychiatrist who had turned his back on psychoanalysis and was appointed as chair of the taskforce that had to develop the third edition of the *DSM* – wanted to change all this. And he did. Thereby, one could say, he fulfilled the dream of Emil Kraepelin, the 'Linnaeus of psychiatry', a dream which was not only about establishing a system of mental disease entities, but also about linking the psychic to the somatic (or neurological) dimension. In 1883 Kraepelin wrote: 'The inner connection between cerebral and psychic functions for us so far has been physiologically absolutely incomprehensible, in truth we know only this, that it anyhow exists and in all probability is a systematic one' (Dillmann 1990: 95).[19] Exactly this assertive uncertainty, or uncertain assertiveness, permeates the global mental health regime that was initiated with the launch of *DSM-III*. And the pharmaceutical industry, as we know today, tapped into this ambiguity rather cunningly and successfully.

Spitzer, as Shorter reports, was more a researcher than a clinician (Shorter 2013: 131). Research orientedness therefore characterized the revolutionary edition that the taskforce leader started to develop with his team. At first Spitzer chose team members 'who were committed primarily to medically oriented, diagnostic research and not to clinical practice', clinicians with nonmedical backgrounds were included later in the process, 'but only after the *DSM-III*'s medically oriented and symptom-focused ground rules had been set' (Mayes and Horwitz 2005: 259). The primary choice, in other words, was for Kraepelinians instead of Freudians. Kraepelin's approach at the time had been based on three main ideas:

> that mental disorders are best understood as analogues with physical diseases; that the classification of mental disorders demands careful observation of visible symptoms instead of on inferences based on unproven causal theories; and that empirical research will eventually demonstrate the organic and biochemical origins of mental disorders.
>
> Ibid.: 260

In that spirit, Spitzer worked on his antipsychoanalytic 'counterrevolution' (Shorter 1997: 300). His bottom line was: 'mental disorders are a subset of medical disorders'. That controversial line did not make it to the final version of *DSM-III*, but clearly expresses Spitzer's inclination, his 'positivistic drive' (Mayes and Horwitz 2005: 260f).[20]

However, a positivist scientific spirit was not the only thing driving this manual, it was, in many ways, also a highly political document, serving the interests of various parties (ibid.: 263).[21] This new, neo-Kraepelinian, standardized system was warmly welcomed by the group of increasingly influential research-oriented psychiatrists, who assumed measurements of mental illness would gain in reliability and validity; practising clinicians, whose claims to treat real diseases were now legitimized; insurance companies, which wanted to see the intangible psychodynamic continuum replaced by a system of discrete disease categories; pharmaceutical companies, which now were provided with clear targets for their product development; and, last but not least, patients, who could now identify with a real disease and seemed to get help more easily (ibid.: 250ff).[22] Mental disorder, in sum, had suddenly become a much more tangible and controllable thing.

DSM rules

The tide had turned. The conceptual shift heralded a revolution in mental health care practice. The little-used *DSM-II* transformed into the biblical *DSM-III*. By the mid-1980s the transition in the USA from a dynamic psychosocial model to a static biopsychiatric symptom-oriented view of mental health was complete (Mayes and Horwitz 2005: 264). With the arrival of *DSM-III*, biomedical researchers had taken the place of clinicians as the most influential voices in the mental health discourse. The basic assumption of the neo-Kraepelinians was that primary symptoms of mental disorders are rooted in a specific form of brain dysfunction (Mayes and Horwitz 2005: 265). In 1989 president George Bush officially sealed this footing by declaring the coming decennium to be the 'Decade of the Brain' (ibid.: 263). The stage was set for the rise of 'Big Pharma'.[23]

Thanks to the anti-psychiatric movement – which had combatted the psychoanalytically stimulated pathologization of normality[24] – and the positivist counterrevolution – which had reawakened the spirit of Kraepelin – the identity crisis that had marked American psychiatry since the mid-1960s had come to an end, at the expense of dynamic psychiatry (ibid.: 252). A new 'scientific' psychiatry came to the fore. And this new view then would conquer the world. The international impact of *DSM-III* and the revised edition *DSM-III-TR* of 1987 was immense. By the early 1990s the manual had been translated into more than 20 languages. 'In Germany, the translation of *DSM-III-TR* reawakened Kraepelinian memories of psychiatric "diseases" (*Krankheiten*) and not just "disorders"' (Shorter 1997: 302). Why, then, still this term 'disorder' in the title of the manual? That caution, one could say, is part of the (neo)Kreapelinian double-dealing, its strategic coupling of uncertainty and assertiveness. In the words of Shorter: 'Even though the drafters shunned the

Kraepelinian label "disease", at the bottom identifying distinct "disorders" meant distinct disease entities' (ibid.: 303).

For Shorter the *DSM* finished a development that started around the turn of the nineteenth to the twentieth century: that of a gradual shift from 'nerves' to 'mood disorder'. The final blow to the nervous syndrome was the separation by the *DSM-III* taskforce of depression and anxiety. In the 1960s and 1970s mixed anxiety-depression – according to Shorter 'the true inheritor of nerves' – was still very much alive (Shorter 2013: 118ff).[25] In September 1974 *DSM-III* chair Spitzer decided to separate the team that dealt with depression from that which dealt with anxiety. It was a disastrous decision, says Shorter, 'they did not know what they were doing' (Shorter 2013: 132).

Depression, formally separated now by the 'disease-designers'(ibid.: 66) from anxiety and no longer bearing the psychoanalytical stamp of neurosis[26] – categorized as one of the 'affective disorders' and carrying the label of 'major depression' – would henceforth be on the up and up in the late modern discourse on mental health. Shorter links this rise of the depression diagnosis mainly to what he terms 'neurotransmitter chatter' and 'a media psychocircus of suggestion' (ibid.: 152, Shorter 1997: 323). It did not have anything to do, he writes, with the introduction of the so-called 'new antidepressants' like Prozac being much more effective than the older drugs. They were not. The 'green medicine' – that is, the barbiturates – were already quite successful: 'The evidence for the effectiveness of the barbiturates for depression and anxiety is considerable,' as opposed to the lack of proof, cleverly concealed, for the positive effect of the new drugs (Shorter 2013: 150). What had prevented depression before from becoming epidemic in the USA was the dominant psychiatric climate: psychoanalytically trained psychiatrists were not 'into' depression and were reluctant in prescribing medications (ibid.: 151). After the neo-Kraepelinian revolution this could change. And it did.

The machinations of Big Pharma were not the only reason why this happened. According to Shorter, it was also a matter of self-preservation of psychiatry as a discipline. To maintain itself against nonmedical competition, against which the medical profession was less and less formally protected, and responding to an increasing demand for psychological services, psychiatry chose to broaden the disease categories – for instance, that of depression. The pharmaceutical industry capitalized on this, 'shifting the focus from disease to unhappiness' (Shorter 1997: 292) very successfully – for instance, via researchers who presented fluoxetine – later baptized Prozac – as an effective drug for a whole range of disorders, which they suggested then could be conceptually classified as affective spectrum disorder (ASD). These researchers, so Shorter quotes, around 1990 began to speak of depression as one of 'the most widespread diseases of mankind' and of ASD as affecting 'possibly one third of the population of the world' (ibid.: 323). A 'media psychocircus of suggestion' subsequently made sure that the hypothesis seemed to be a natural law, which made people in massive numbers ask for help because of a 'mood disorder' (ibid.). These people, Shorter emphatically states again and again, are not ill but unhappy. But, if so, one may wonder why. Why is this sort of 'unhappiness' so widespread today? Is there some kind of collective discontent in late modern culture at stake? Do we need to speak in terms of social or cultural pathology here? These sort of questions, however, are not part of Shorter's agenda.

They are absent too in the work that is frequently quoted in texts on the so-called depression epidemic, *The Loss of Sadness: How Psychiatry Transformed Normal Sorrow into Depressive Disorder* (2007), by sociologist Allan V. Horwitz and philosopher/social scientist Jerome C. Wakefield. The authors, as the subtitle already indicates, focus on the pathologization of 'normal sorrow', that is to say 'sadness' which is simply part of life. Like Shorter, they see the publication of *DSM-III* in 1980 as a turning point, 'a watershed in the history of psychiatric diagnosis' (Horwitz and Wakefield 2007: 97). Here ended 2,500 years of psychiatry, they state, during which 'normal human nature' was taken as something that includes 'a propensity to potentially intense sadness after certain kinds of loss' (ibid.: 87). Traditionally it was acknowledged that mental disorder should be understood in terms of its specific context, or, in other words, in terms of the proportionality of the link between cause and intensity or duration of symptoms. Sadness is normal and presumably has protective functions – which, according to the authors, are still not properly understood (ibid.: 23) – but becomes pathological, that is destructive, when the response to a loss is disproportionate to the nature of the latter. For this situation Horwitz and Wakefield use the term 'harmful dysfunction' (ibid.: 17).[27] They take into account that 'proportionality' is also a culturally informed thing, but emphasize that the underlying mechanism is not. So sadness as a response to loss is either 'design or dysfunction': there is normal sadness because of the functioning of a biologically designed loss response mechanism, or there is pathological sadness because of the malfunctioning of this mechanism (ibid.: 46). The disaster of the *DSM-III* turn, the two social scientists assert, consists in the elimination of this contextual view. The symptoms were decontextualized and became free-floating. And, because of that, the fairly clear distinction between normal and pathological sadness became a very blurred one.

Two years before *The Loss of Sadness*, and in collaboration with political scientist Rick Mayes, Horwitz published an excellent article – to which I have already referred a few times – entitled '*DSM-III* and the revolution in the classification of mental illness', in which the major shift in psychiatry of 1980 is placed into its context. *DSM-III*, they write, 'radically transformed the nature of mental illness' (Mayes and Horwitz 2005: 250). A medical model was introduced in psychiatry, which made diagnosis – that is, discriminating discrete disease entities – the mainstay of psychiatric research and clinical practice. How could this happen? Why was this shift of *DSM-III* such a tremendous success? What transformed the *DSM* from a fairly unpopular local guide into a global canonical text? For this, there are three possible explanations, Mayes and Horwitz write. One is that it was a victory of reason, a triumph of science, an injection of a positivist spirit into psychiatry, which, according to many, was still way too 'metaphysically' inspired. Suddenly objectivity seemed to be in close range. In the USA, the turn of 1980 was widely celebrated like this (Shorter 1997: 302). A second common explanation of the success of *DSM-III* is that it was at the heart of a growing movement of medicalization of mental malaises. The number of diagnoses from *DSM-I* to *DSM-III* had almost tripled, the number of pages almost quadrupled, which was seen as evidence of psychiatry's growing legitimized power to classify and treat mental problems as medical ones. The third explanation – and this is the one Mayes and Horwitz opt for – is that the key to the success of *DSM-III* is its focus on categorical, symptom-based diagnosis in defining mental disorders.

> In contrast to the position that these diagnoses represented the growth of scientific knowledge, we argue that no new knowledge led to the new paradigm. Likewise, although the *DSM-III* did greatly increase the number of specific diagnoses, it did not increase the number of behaviors that psychiatry laid claim to treat. Psychoanalysis had already medicalized a vast number of problems over the course of the twentieth century.
>
> Mayes and Horwitz 2005: 251

So, *DSM-III* didn't expand the range of treatable problems, but only redefined these into discrete disease entities. Mental malaise suddenly had become a tangible thing. And this, as said earlier, served the interests of various parties involved.

Is this sadness, is this normal?

Although elucidating, there are some problems with these analyses of Horwitz & Co. Considering their definition of depression as sadness that is disproportionate to its cause, Matthew Ratcliffe points out in *Experiences of Depression* that it is unclear how (dis)proportionateness should be determined because it depends on cultural and personal evaluations that may be implicit, ambivalent or ambiguous. Moreover, writes Ratcliffe, causal links between depression and life events are hard to establish; cause and effect are often intertwined. Furthermore, and for us here most importantly, depression is not simply a matter of extreme sadness (Ratcliffe 2015: 265). There is more, and often sadness is not prominent or even absent. The heart of depression, so my thesis is here, is not sadness but a fundamental feeling of isolation; it involves, in the words of Ratcliffe, the disruption of a basic 'sense of belonging' or 'existential trust'. I will return to this central idea shortly.

First, back to Horwitz & Co.'s contextualization of the 'decontextualization of mental disorder'. *DSM-III* most certainly involved a shift towards 'hard science' – that is, positivism, so towards more immediate tangibility, an ostensible tangibility, of course, which nevertheless appeared as 'real'. And it surely also meant intensified medicalization or pathologization of individual suffering, in the sense of becoming more efficient, specific, targeted, due to a switch from a presupposed continuum to a system of distinct entities, which – like

Kraepelin almost a century earlier already suggested – cannot be established yet as entities, but are expected to be substantiated someday. Whether this, indeed, will happen can be doubted. But it need not happen because the *DSM* system already functions 'effectively', it functions *on the basis* of its promise, its assertive uncertainty or uncertain assertiveness.

Horwitz & Co. seem to take the decontextualization of mental disorder – like Shorter does with the reduction of the 'nervous syndrome' – as a sort of accidental mistake and the outcomes of it as a kind of collateral damage, damage that can be repaired by focusing on the concept of 'harmful dysfunction'. In *The Loss of Sadness* it is stated that the so-called depression epidemic, 'although the result of many social factors', is 'largely a product of conflating the two conceptually distinct categories of normal sadness and depressive disorder'. To which the authors add: 'there are no obvious circumstances that would explain a recent upsurge in depressive disorder', no such 'environmental pathogen' has been 'identified or even theorized' (Horwitz and Wakefield 2007: 6f).

That was in 2007. Many sensible words had already been spoken then about a possible 'environmental pathogen' of depression. Nine years earlier, French sociologist Alain Ehrenberg had written *La Fatigue d'Être Soi. Dépression et Société*,[28] in which he analysed the rise of the diagnosis of depression in late modern civilization in terms of the establishment of a new postneurotic normativity and subjectivity. The late modern subject, Ehrenberg explained, is a *homo economicus* – that is, an enterprising subject, a 'Me Ltd', and depression is the flipside of it. In the book that can be considered the prequel of this first volume in the series The Social Pathologies of Contemporary Civilization, a book with the same title as this series, I paraphrased Ehrenberg's analysis as follows:

> Late modernity is not dominated anymore by prohibition but by incitement. What is expected from the individual is not restriction and sublimation but mobilization and expression of his passions. Henceforth the thing is to get the most out of oneself. One needs to 'be oneself' and become it even more. One must show initiative, motivation, determination, purposefulness, versatility and communicability. Human despondency thus is no longer understood in terms of conflict and guilt, but of defect and shame. Depression in this context appears as failure in what is being called for. Being depressed means not being able or willing to have a project, be enterprising, assertive, on the move. It means being unwilling or unable to realize oneself. Depression, in Ehrenberg's words, is 'the disease of responsibility', or 'the fatigue of becoming oneself'.
>
> Bergh 2013: 91–2

Two years before *The Loss of Sadness* German sociologist Hartmut Rosa had published *Beschleunigung. Die Veränderung der Zeitstrukturen in der Moderne*,[29] in which he explained one of the big paradoxes of late modern life: technology and prosperity have provided us with an abundance of time, but we experience a growing lack of it. He tackles this paradox by analysing the processes of social acceleration that are involved in modern times. The process of acceleration is an integral part of modernity, Rosa writes, but has become destructive in late modernity – that is, in the last 30 or 40 years, so since about 1980. In the above-mentioned chapter I outlined Rosa's argument as follows:

> This process has reached a point after which the claim to social synchronization and integration no longer can be substantiated. The consequence of this is a fundamental shift in the forms of social control and individual self-relation: these become 'situative', that is to say, they are determined each time anew on the basis of the context concerned. One lives 'in the moment', in a present that tends to shrink because it is less and less destined by the past and tailored to the future, since the past has lost its binding power and the future is experienced as utterly unpredictable.
>
> Bergh 2013: 93

From Rosa's perspective, then, the late modern subject is a *homo mobilis*, with a 'situative' identity, having increasingly intense difficulties with synchronizing his life with and integrating it into a meaningful whole. This leads to a collective basic experience of 'raging standstill', which turns pathological as clinical depression. This disorder Rosa therefore considers – like Ehrenberg – to be the main malaise of contemporary civilization. He terms depression the 'pathology of time', which means …

> firstly: the key disorder of late modernity, secondly: an outcome of the time pressure that marks this epoch, and thirdly: a sensation of stagnation and futurelessness which announces itself in the middle of all dynamism. If we look upon depression like that, the depressed person no longer appears merely as 'disturbed' or 'disordered' but acquires the status of most sensitive seismograph of present and coming transformations.
>
> Ibid., 94

The big question, then, is what kind of sensitivity is at stake here.

And, finally, four years before the publication of Horwitz and Wakefield's classic, French philosopher Dany-Robert Dufour started his analysis of what he called the 'liberal cultural revolution' with a book that had the telling title *L'Art de Réduire les Têtes. Sur la nouvelle servitude de l'homme libérale à l'ère du capitalisme total* (2003).[30] Like Ehrenberg and Rosa, Dufour makes a sharp distinction between modernity and post- or late modernity – as also expounded in Chapter 2 of this volume. In the shift from the former to the latter era an 'anthropological mutation' has taken place, that is 'a radical transformation of our subjective condition' (Dufour 2008: 5, 13, this volume, Ch. 2). Because of the loss of 'the Other' or the 'big Subject', the late modern subject has become completely self-referential, confronted with the impossible task of self-foundation, mobilized by and responding to the 'Divine Market', which presents itself as a new big Subject, but is fully inadequate to be such, so Dufour states in Chapter 2, 'because it has nothing to offer the subject on the problem of foundation'. Earlier, in *The Art of Shrinking Heads*, he wrote: 'Exchanges are no longer valid insofar as they are guaranteed by some higher power (either transcendental or ethical); they are valid by virtue of the direct relationship they establish as commodities. Commodity exchanges are, in a word, beginning to desymbolize the world.' And: 'Human beings no longer have to agree about transcendent symbolic values; they simply have to go along with the never-ending and expanded circulation of commodities' (Dufour 2008: 4f). To which I added, in 'Depression: resisting ultra-liberalism?':

> This pliability, cloaked as self-fulfilment, makes us go adrift. The former modern subject, who had a critical and neurotic nature – two characteristics that complemented each other perfectly according to Dufour – transformed into a creature that smoothly fits in with the flows and pulses of the global market. Dufour speaks of 'a precarious, acritical, psychotisizing subject' and specifies the latter term as follows: 'by psychotisizing I mean a subject that is open to all identity fluctuations and thereby is susceptible to all commercial bifurcations'.
>
> Bergh 2013: 88

Deinstitutionalization and desymbolization – or, in one word, decontextualization – are two sides of the same 'neoliberal' coin, and this coin pays off as the 'psychotization', that is to say the destabilizing sensitization of the subject. The global market of 'total capitalism', Dufour states in *The Art of Shrinking Heads*, destroys institutions and reshapes procedures 'in such a way as to produce individuals who are supple, insecure, mobile and open to all the market's modes and variations' (Dufour 2008: 157).

Dufour's analysis of the gradual historical process of liberation of the human passions – which, for him, makes up the heart of 'liberalism' – reveals it as a process that started with Blaise Pascal and moved via, among others, Bernard de Mandeville, Adam Smith and Marquis De Sade to the contemporary world of dynamized production and eroticized consumption, a world inhabited by a pliable and susceptible flexi-worker/trend-follower, who all along and on all sides is incited to realize the liberal phantasy that De Sade staged in literary space more than two centuries ago, a phantasy of an 'isolist' – that is, an extremely egoistic and hedonistic subject. De Sade's phantasy is our reality. 'We live in an increasingly Sadean world,' Dufour writes in *La Cité Perverse* (Dufour 2009: 11).[31] And, in Chapter 2 of the present volume, he states: 'we have moved from a mostly symbolic to a mostly libidinal functioning'. The late modern subjectification of the *homo economicus/homo mobilis* turns the modern subject into a *homo libidinosus*: an 'isolist' or 'Sadean' subject whose passions are liberated in order to be colonized and mobilized by the 'Divine Market'.

Through the 1980s, after the 'liberating' 1960s and 1970s, the mobilization of the passions gained momentum. The rise of 'neoliberalism' – which from a

Dufourian angle could also be termed 'ultraliberalism' – was, at the same time, the dawn of the 'Prozac era'. The mental disorder depression became a hot potato. This happened for 'internal' reasons, as discussed by Shorter and Horwitz & Co., but also, more fundamentally, for 'contextual' reasons, as analysed by Ehrenberg, Rosa and Dufour. Is the depressive 'strategy', as Dufour calls it in Chapter 2 of this volume, perhaps a protective move, as Horwitz and Wakefield suggested in *The Loss of Sadness*, adding that the 'healing and reparative functions' of depression 'are still not understood'? (Horwitz and Wakefield 2007: 23). But can we really understand the depressive 'strategy' without taking a phenomenological perspective? Obviously, I don't think we can. 'Our situation calls for a phenomenology of depression,' I wrote in 'Depression: resisting ultra-liberalism?' (Bergh 2013: 98). To the perspective of the Belgian 'pathoanalist' Jacques Schotte that was presented there, from which depression needs to be understood in terms of 'attunement' and 'distunement' at a 'pre-intentional, pre-subjective, participative level' (ibid.), I would like to add here two similar perspectives: that of the British philosopher Matthew Ratcliffe, already indicated, who recently published *Experiences of Depression: A Study in Phenomenology* (2015), in which depression is discussed as a 'existential change' involving a corrosion or loss of a 'sense of belonging'; and that of the German psychiatrist Thomas Fuchs, who has written several phenomenologically inspired texts in which depression comes to the fore as a disorder of 'intersubjective time', 'interaffectivity', 'intercorporeality' and thus as a process or dynamic state of 'detunement' at a very basic affective level.

In one of these texts Fuchs writes: 'Phenomenology precisely offers a way to regain access to this pre-reflective dimension of experience, namely through methodically "bracketing" our culture-bound and science-based assumptions about the nature and causes of affective experience' (Fuchs 2013: 226; cf Ratcliffe 2015: 19ff). This 'bracketing' – the classical phenomenological *epoché* – concerns, among other things, our present *DSM*-inspired understanding of depression, or, in other words, the *epoché* has to be executed on depression as a cultural syndrome. In that way we might get to understand more about what is at stake in the experience of depression, what its particular 'unhappiness' and possible 'protective functions' are about. Via such a phenomenological move the state of isolation that was discussed at the beginning of this chapter could be meaningfully linked with the isolist condition of the late modern 'Sadean' subject. Is the so-called depression epidemic above all a devastating confrontation with the 'Sadean' position? And is this confrontation, at the same time, directly or indirectly, an awakening or reawakening of that which is warded off, corroded or lost in this position: the 'inter' of 'interaffectivity', 'intercorporeality' and 'intersubjectivity' Fuchs speaks about, or the 'sym' of the 'sympathetic' individualism that, according to Dufour, may arrive 'after liberalism'?

Anthropology calls

But before we take up these questions, we need to get back again to the 1980s because, in those years, another important development took place – a development that directly touches upon the line of argumentation put forward in this chapter – namely the rise of cross-cultural or transcultural, or simply cultural psychiatry and psychology. So, on the one hand, as discussed above, these years were marked by the neo-Kraepelinian revolution, the turn to biopsychiatry and the emergence of Big Pharma. The *DSM* regime started to colonize mental health care all over the world. On the other hand, however, being the aftermath of decolonization and the heyday of multiculturalism, these years were marked by an intensified call from the field of anthropology to give more attention to the role of culture in the constitution of mental disorders. The 1980s, then seem to have been a matter of a growing opposition between a 'universalist' biopsychiatry and a 'relativist' anthropology. This opposition, however, although clearly the case, needs to be put in its proper perspective too. First, it was, surprisingly enough, the godfather of biopsychiatry himself, Emil Kraepelin, who at the beginning of the twentieth century, after a study trip to Ceylon, India, Singapore and Indonesia, published an article in the authoritative *Centralblatt für Nervenheilkunde und Psychiatrie* (1904) in which he pleaded for a new subdiscipline, namely that of '*Vergleichende Psychiatrie*', comparative psychiatry, which should focus on ethnic and socio-cultural aspects of mental health and disease. So from the start, one could say, biopsychiatry at least was sensitive to cultural differences. But Kraepelin's death in 1926 also meant the dying away of the call for a cross-cultural psychiatry (Jilek 1995: 237; cf Jilek 2014). It was only 35 years later that this branch of psychiatry started to flourish, when 'ethnic psychiatry' or 'exotic psychiatry' turned into 'transcultural psychiatry'; an unquestioned ethnocentric perspective gradually made way for a view that acknowledged the need to build conceptual bridges to other cultures. But the real acknowledgement of cultural differences substantiated around 1980, when the term 'cultural psychiatry' became current and the ethnocentric character of *every* perspective was taken into account (Tseng *et al.* 2014: 18).[32]

Furthermore, anthropological relativism does not necessarily exclude universalism. I turn now to a watershed collection of anthropological and cross-cultural studies on depression which was published five years after the revolution of *DSM-III*, entitled *Culture and Depression: Studies in the Anthropology and Cross-cultural Psychiatry of Affect and Disorder*, edited by anthropologist/psychiatrist Arthur Kleinman and anthropologist Byron Good (1985). The key thought in this collection is that of a basic psychosomatic process which, via the 'work of culture', takes shape into a concrete phenomenon.[33] So a universal underlying process is culturally formed into a culture-specific experience, which, concerning what in the West is termed 'depression', might be considered a disorder, or might not, and which might be understood in similar ways as in western mental health views, or might not. Within the perspective of this collection of studies the famous idea of 'somatization' as 'masked depression', for instance, is refuted: both 'somatization' and 'psychologization' are specific outcomes of the 'work of culture'.[34] I will come back to this latter issue hereafter, highlighting three central thoughts of *Culture and Depression*.

I called this work a watershed collection because it is at the heart of the turning point from 'transcultural psychiatry' to 'cultural psychiatry', it is permeated with a call to give more attention to the role of culture in the constitution of mental disorders. Being the outcome of a double panel at the American Anthropological Association (AAA) Annual Meeting in 1982, in this collection we find an assembly of scholars who are worried about the consequences of the neo-Kraepelinian revolution which just had taken place: 'there is a growing consensus in the psychiatric community that the current criteria of depression are valid and represent criteria of a universal, biologically grounded disease'. And this unfounded certainty, the editors continue, 'provokes anthropological response' (Kleinman and Good 1985: 5).[35] In the Epilogue of the book Kleinman and Good repeat again the main thought of the collection: 'Depressive illness and dysphoria are thus not only interpreted differently in non-Western societies and across cultures; they are *constituted* as fundamentally different forms of social reality.' As a 'social reality', depression calls for 'a theoretical perspective that is thoroughly interactionist' (ibid.: 492). And there we have the three key ideas of *Culture and Depression* I want to highlight here: first, depression as constituted by the 'work of culture', second, depression as a 'social affect' or 'drama' and, third, 'somatization' as well as 'psychologization' as culture-specific shapings or 'stagings' of a primordial universal process, whereby 'somatization' is the rule rather than the exception.[36]

'Depression' – or however the dysphoria is culturally termed – as a *social* phenomenon, a 'social affect', understood in terms of a basic 'attunement', is a key thought in two texts on depression of the already mentioned Jacques Schotte, which he wrote around the same time as *Culture and Depression* was conceived and which I paraphrased in 'Depression: resisting ultra-liberalism?' (Bergh 2013). That was 30 years ago. It seems that only recently this kind of phenomenological interpretation has started gaining momentum in the work of people like Thomas Fuchs and Matthew Ratcliffe.

Connecting the issues raised in *Culture and Depression* with the 'environmental pathogens' discussed in the former section, one could say, using the distinction Arthur and Joan Kleinman make between the 'social production of disease' and the 'cultural construction of illness' (Kleinman and Good 1985: 466ff), that the analysis of Ehrenberg concerns the latter, whereas that of Rosa touches the former. Depression is 'staged' in late modern culture as the flipside of the dominant normativity of self-realization. The context in which this 'drama' takes place is that of social acceleration, which has become disruptive, leading to all sorts of integration issues and synchronization problems. The 'situative' identity of the late modern subject, as Rosa terms it, is philosophically deepened by Dufour, who in his historical analysis traces the Sadean, 'isolist' subject back to Pascal, the first 'perverse puritan', who initiated the inversion or perversion of the Augustinian hierarchy of *Amor Dei* and *amor sui*, divine love and self-love – leading eventually to the self-referential subject of neo- or ultraliberalism, for which *amor sui* is the main road to glory (Bergh 2013: 88ff). Thinking in these terms, one could take the 'depression epidemic' as the collective confrontation with the 'Sadean' position, as the common-but-not-shared isolation of 'isolism'. However, in order to get to understand what exactly is disrupted there, and in what way, one needs, as Fuchs states, to 'bracket' the present common sense on depression, informed by 'neoliberalism' and '*DSM* regime', in order to gain access to the 'pre-reflective dimension of experience', the primordial sphere of 'interaffectivity', 'intercorporeality' and 'sympathy', where a disturbance of a basic attunement, so a 'detunement' or 'distunement', takes place.[37]

The phenomenological maxim of getting back to the *Sache selbst*,[38] means regaining access to what has become unspeakable. In order to 'retrieve the hidden layers of our own experience', Fuchs writes, we need to 'change our concepts' (Fuchs 2013: 226). The 'burden' of depression is 'hidden', depression is 'taboo', not so much because we turn away from it or keep silent about it, but rather because it is ineffable because we lack the proper narrative for it. We need to turn away from the 'individualistic', or, more specifically, the 'neoliberal' or 'ultraliberal' conception of subjectivity and connected ideas of 'the good life'. We need to retap into the tradition of phenomenology and get back to the matter itself – that is, the primordial pre-reflective, pre-intentional, pre-subjective level of (inter)affective, (inter)corporeal *attunement*. Inspiration to do so, Fuchs points out, can come from the field of anthropology, where affect often appears to be much more socially defined and experienced (ibid.: 225). What we often find in other cultures as well, is the experience of illness as that of an integral sociopsychosomatic unity. The Eurocentric split between *soma* and *psyche* keeps us from understanding these 'exotic' experiences, but also, and this is the phenomenological bottom line here, from understanding our own experiences of depression (ibid.: 221). What is painfully lacking in psychiatry, Fuchs states – and one could add: what is lacking overall in the present dominant discourse on mental health and pathology – is a concept of the 'lived body' and of the 'organic unity of the embodied person'. The disaster of the traditional dualism of mind and body has only been worsened by its shifting towards a reductionist monism, 'which now regards the brain as the true heir of the soul'. What we need and what phenomenology can offer is an 'ecological, non-reductionist view of depression' (ibid.: 234). A whole body of work is waiting for us, inspired by Heidegger, Merleau-Ponty and others: Tellenbach's *Melancholie*,[39] the work of Schotte, Fuchs, Ratcliffe and much more.[40]

Conclusion: towards a post-Sadean education

In *Culture and Depression*, the Singhalese anthropologist Gananath Obeyesekere refers to the definition that Brown and Harris used in their famous study on the social sources of depression, as being in the core 'generalized hopelessness', to which he remarks: 'This statement sounds strange to me, a Buddhist, for if it was placed in the context of Sri Lanka, I would say that we are not dealing with a depressive but a good Buddhist', for which 'hopelessness lies in the nature of the world, and salvation lies in understanding and overcoming that hopelessness' (Kleinman and Good 1985: 134, cf 467).[41] Buddhism offers a framework for reflection on hopelessness or despair, something which, according to Obeyesekere, is missing in western society, wherein depressive affects 'are not anchored to an ideology and are therefore identifiable and conducive to labelling as illness' (ibid.: 135). If we apply this remark to our present situation, we might say: not 'anchored' perhaps, but there is indeed an 'ideology' which frames these affects, as analysed by Ehrenberg, contextualized by Rosa and philosophically deepened by Dufour – the ultraliberal 'ideology' of a self-referential, self-realizing, hyperdynamic, hyperflexible, situative, isolist subject, in brief a Sadean subject, constantly exposed to and mobilized by an omnipresent Sadean education. We need to find ways of resisting that. We are in need of a post-Sadean education, or, in Rosa's terms, a *Resonanzpädagogik* (Rosa and Endres 2016). In order to come to that, however, we first need to understand what this 'attunement' is that makes the 'resonance' possible. Or, conversely, in the spirit of Schotte's 'pathoanalysis' – in which one unlocks the sources of human existence via the analysis of pathology – we need to know what kind of primordial 'distunement' is involved in the phenomenon we tend to term 'depression'. Or, in other words again, those of Fuchs, we need to refind a conceptualization of the 'lived body'.

I would like to return one last time to *Culture and Depression*, to the issue discussed there by Kleinman and Kleinman of 'somatization' versus 'psychologization'; the idea of depression as 'drama' – that is, a specific 'staging' of a basic sociopsychosomatic reality – comes to the fore here in a clarifying manner. Both 'somatization' and 'psychologization', one could say, are masked manifestations of depression, in the sense that the socio-cultural context forces this basic reality in a certain direction, which led in China, as the Kleinmans show, to an 'idiom of bodily complaints and medical helpseeking' and in the West – but only since Victorian times – to an 'increasingly psychological idiom of distress' (Kleinman and Good 1985: 434). In the late 1970s and early 1980s, when the research the Kleinmans report on was being conducted, depression in China was still constructed as 'neurasthenia', entailing a focus on so-called vegetative symptoms, that is 'sleep, appetite, energy, cognitive and sexual disturbance, and psychomotor retardation or agitation', plus a close link to anxiety disorders. The background of this, so the Kleinmans explain, is a certain traditional stigma connected with the expression of dysphoria in China, a stigma which was heavily radicalized during Mao's cultural revolution: dysphoria meant dissent, and the 'staging' of depression as neurasthenia was, so to say, politically correct (ibid.: 436f).

Now it might be elucidating to look at the depression alarm which is sounding presently on all sides in western societies in light of the above-mentioned political correctness. What exactly is threatened in late modern civilization, being the final stage of the 'liberal cultural revolution'? How is depression staged today? What is our present political correctness? What turn did the 'psychologization' of depression take? It is certainly a complicated issue, or maybe one should say a split one, for whereas, on the one hand, depression is classified as an affective disorder and linked to neurobiological malfunctioning, on the other hand, in therapeutic settings cognitive models are often applied, with cognitive behaviour therapy as the absolute favourite (Fuchs 2013: 220). In both approaches the 'lived body' is far off. And in both approaches the remobilization of the depressed person – with 'resilience' as a key term – appears to be the main aim. The threat of late modern depression is that of the unproductivity, immobility, insensitivity – in one word, immobilizability – of the subject. Could depression then, indeed, be a sort of retreat from this and thus the expression of a sort of discontent? If so, it seems to be a rather helpless one.

Resisting the Sadean education means regaining access to what is referred to by Schotte as 'primary passion': 'primary passion of the soul, through which this soul starts to appear in the world, to the others, and via these to itself' (Schotte 1982: 667). It is the sphere in which a *pré-moi participatif*, a participative presubject, is involved in a process of continuous reciprocal attunement with an *ambiance*, which Schotte relates to the ancient Greek word *periechon*, meaning something like the encompassing bearing, so not something that is surrounding an already constituted subject but something which constitutes the presubject into a subject while this presubject is already resonating to that ambiance (ibid.: 648). It is a sphere of primordial participation, an affective being-in-the-world before any subject/object opposition: 'a sort of reciprocal interiority of "self" and a world constituted by others as well, who together with this "self" (re)find themselves already on their way in the coming-and-going and the general anonymity of a primary participation' (ibid.: 668). This primordial attunement can turn into a distunement or detunement when the 'feeling presubject' has problems with 'participating productively-receptively in the global ambient coming-and-going of nature and life' (ibid.: 643, 638). So the 'mood disorder' depression is basically a participation disorder, as also Fuchs acknowledges: 'the patients lose the participation in the shared space of affective attunement', or, in the words of Ratcliffe, it involves a loss or corrosion of 'a changeable sense of belonging to the world that is pre-subjective and pre-objective' (Fuchs 2013: 228; Ratcliffe 2015: 56). Ratcliffe terms this disruption of the sense of belonging as 'existential change', thereby redefining depression into an existential phenomenon: 'the label "depression" could be restricted to cases that involve existential changes'. The so-called depression epidemic would then involve different variants of 'existential depression' (Ratcliffe 2015: 253).

Schotte took depression as the central disorder of psychiatry, he called it 'the most ubiquitously important one of the whole of psychiatry in the practice of medicine in general, and as having played therefore its frequent paradigm-role in the history of psychiatry' (Schotte 1989: 79). The 'pathoanalysis' of depression leads directly to the basis of human existence, the intangible sphere of basic interwovenness, of primordial contact, which is described by Schotte in musical terms, with words like 'tone' and 'rhythm': a correspondence is executed 'according to the tone of a situation and according to the rhythm of an exchange which already on this elementary-primordial "level" can realize themselves as harmonious or, on the contrary, be analysed as more or less disharmonious' (Schotte 1982: 623, 673). This disharmony or distunement involves a 'slackening of all functions of resonance as well as exchange' (ibid.: 669). The Belgian pathoanalist uses three Latin terms to typify depression: *anhormia*, lack of drive or zest; *anhedonia*, lack of interest or pleasure; and *arrhythmia*, disturbance of the rhythm of life (Schotte 1989: 72). One is distuned and therefore disinterested and displeasured. The pre-intentional disruption disturbs intentional relations, and also the self-relation becomes problematic. One is 'stuck'. It is a state of 'alienation', to use Rosa's term (Rosa 2010, 2012, 2016).[42] Ratcliffe speaks of 'estrangement' (Ratcliffe 2015: 202ff). There is a disruption of a basic 'sense of belonging' or 'existential trust'. Therefore, Ratcliffe writes, personal accounts of depression so frequently refer to 'feelings of being vulnerable, exposed, threatened, or unsafe' (ibid.: 220). Ratcliffe also quotes William James, who in *Varieties of Religious Experience*, in the chapter entitled 'The sick soul', speaks of 'the world as fundamentally evil, a place in which we can never be safe or feel at home' (ibid.: 271). The evil of the world is the loss of its inviting and sheltering nature. One no longer feels at home there, one no longer belongs there. One is homeless and aimless. One is isolated.

'Well done!' De Sade calls out then. 'Come to us!' the Market joins in. Neoliberalism or ultraliberalism involves the continuous corrosion of 'existential trust' in order to make the isolist subject mobilizable. There are two common responses to the omnipresent Sadean education to which this subject is continuously exposed: one can throw oneself on the plenitude of offerings of the Market, or one can retreat and radicalize the isolation with the danger of becoming 'depressed'. Is there another possibility? Is there a third way, a way out of this late modern incarcerating condition? In order to find an answer to this question we have to re-educate ourselves. We are desperately in need of an anti-Sadean or post-Sadean education, which involves a redisciplining of the passions, on the basis of a recovery of 'the hidden layers of our own experience' (Fuchs 2013: 226). What we need for our existential renovation, in short, is an education of attunement.

Notes

1 This TV programme intends to be both entertaining and reflective – hence the title, meaning both *The world keeps on turning* and *The world turns mad*.
2 Blue Monday was called into being by the British psychologist Cliff Arnall, as being the most depressing day of the year, on the basis of an alleged scientific formula. In academic circles Arnall's idea is not taken seriously, but via the media it has nevertheless acquired a certain status. Bakker and his fellow organizers of the Depression Gala tied in with this.
3 See NRC 23 January 2016: *Creativiteit is een luxe*; Trouw 25 January 2016: *Extra onderzoek naar depressie jongeren*; de Volkskrant 26 January 2016: *Taboe op depressie breken met 'Depressiegala'*.
4 *With One's Own Hand. Suicide and the Survivors.*
5 From *Darkness Visible* and *Shoot the Damn Dog*.
6 A statement made by Solomon in an interview he had with Zwagerman in 2005 for the Dutch newspaper *Trouw* was quoted frequently after Zwagerman's death: 'Suicide should remain difficult.' The interview was included in three different works of Zwagerman, *Het vijfde seizoen*, *Door eigen hand* and *Americana*.

7 For the term 'Black Dog' as a metaphor for depression, see, for instance, http://www.who.int/mental_health/management/depression/en/ and http://www.blackdoginstitute.org.au/docs/Foley.pdf (accessed 23 June 2016). Just to be clear: not in any way do I pretend here to give an 'explanation' of the suicides referred to at the start of this chapter. Besides a various complex whole of specific personal circumstances, a common factor in these stories is depression, and it is the way this 'problem' is conceived and approached in our late modern society that I focus on here and in my PhD project.

8 In *Depresson und Gesellschaft. Zur Erfindung einer Volkskrankheit* (2012), Konstantin Ingenkamp uses the term 'Depressionsalarmismus' (depression alarmism: 126) to typify the current attitude towards this mental disorder. Depression as we understand it today according to Ingenkamp is a common disease constructed by 'the society of prescribed positive thinking' (335). It is not the outcome but rather the precondition of it. What we need to do therefore, Ingenkamp states at the end of his book, is turn this constructed depression back into 'creative melancholy'. The 'distunement', in other words, should be transformed into a 'retunement'. The key thought in this chapter is that we first need to better understand what 'attunement' entails.

9 http://www.who.int/mental_health/management/depression/en/ (accessed 23 June 2016).

10 *DSM-5* also mentions this 'hidden burden': 'clinicians should be aware that in most countries the majority of cases of depression go unrecognized in primary care settings and that in many cultures, somatic symptoms are very likely to constitute the presenting complaint' (166).

11 Cf: 'a cluster or group of co-occurring, relatively invariant symptoms found in a specific cultural group, community, or context (e.g., *ataque de nervios*). The syndrome may or may not be recognized as an illness within the culture (e.g., it might be labeled in various ways), but such cultural patterns of distress and features of illness may nevertheless be recognizable by an outside observer' (APA 2013: 14).

12 English professor of primary medical care Christopher Dowrick, author of *Beyond Depression* (2009), states in an editorial in a May 2013 issue of the *British Journal of General Practice* that 'depression' seems to fulfil the criteria for a 'culture-bound syndrome' (Dowrick 2013: 229). The term 'culture-bound syndrome' was, in *DSM-5*, replaced by the triad *cultural syndrome/cultural idiom of distress/cultural explanation or perceived cause* (APA 2013: 14).

13 See, for instance, Berrios and Porter 1995: 509–44; Shorter 1997: 129ff, 2013: 31ff; Schuster 2011; Ingenkamp 2012: 131ff; Ehrenberg 1998: 38ff; Ehrenberg 2010a: 49ff.

14 See, for instance, the shift in China from the concept of 'neurasthenia' to that of 'depression' under the influence of the *DSM* regime (Lee 1999).

15 Shorter used this term in a presentation at a conference in Copenhagen in May 2006, published as *The doctrine of the two depressions in historical perspective* in *Acta Psychiatrica Scandinavica* 2007: 115 (Suppl. 433), 5–13. In *How Everyone Became Depressed* he 'specified' nonmelancholic mood disorder as 'nervous syndrome'.

16 Shorter chooses these terms, he explains, to start a discussion, he is 'not entrenched on this'. But a fundamental discussion is urgently needed: 'It is time for a turn-around' (Shorter 2013: 179, 196). There is some confusing use of terms in his text: for instance, separating 'melancholia' from 'nerves' or 'nervous syndrome', but at the same time relating 'melancholia' to 'nervous breakdown'; and whereas Shorter, on the one hand, states that so-called depressed people are not ill, he also speaks of the 'nervous syndrome' as an 'illness' of 'the entire brain and body' that needs to be 'treated' as such. (ibid.88, 198). Cf Shorter and Fink, *Endocrine Psychiatry* (2010), and several texts by others – for instance, in *Acta Psychiatrica Scandinavica* 2007: 115, linked to the above-mentioned Copenhagen symposium in May 2006, Melancholia: Beyond DSM, Beyond Neurotransmitters.

17 Instead of the usual term 'symptomatological'. Although the approach of the *DSM* is labelled as 'categorical', there are, in fact, only classes, not categories. There is no consistent logic in the structure of the text. In the introduction the authors write: 'The organizational structure is meant to serve as a bridge to new diagnostic approaches without disrupting current clinical practice and research' (APA 2013: 13) A shift from 'categorical' to 'dimensional' approaches is announced. The Dutch translation of *DSM-5* (APA 2014) is even more cautious (or modest) than the original text, dropping the adjective 'diagnostic' from the title because, so the translators write in their editorial justification, this word 'has possibly contributed to the overrating of the meaning of the DSM-system'. This system is 'no more, but also no less than an extensive classification system: an overview of the current way in which mental disorders can be classified' (ibid.: 43f). This somewhat peculiar formulation ('current' and 'can') seems to express the ambivalence of the *DSM* project: alleged hypothesis-oriented research spirit versus factual protocol directed clinical practice. For mental health care professionals the *ICD* codes that go along with the *DSM* disorder labels are not connected to a 'can' but to a 'must'. No code – no pay – no cure, so to speak. Could a shift to 'dimensional approaches' take place without replacing the current (neo)Kraepelinian mental health regime as such? Is the announcement of such a shift in the *DSM* – considering the way in which this regime presently functions – really more than an empty promise?

18 See, for instance, Ratcliffe 2015: 3ff, 188, 218; Milders and Thunissen 2015: 69ff. The first work is an attempt to unfold a phenomenology of depression, taken as a heterogeneous category, which nonetheless can be linked to a number of central themes, or, in other words, has 'a degree of phenomenological unity' (71). The second work, written by two experienced Dutch psychiatrists/psychiatric instructors, discusses the 'endangered' status of psychiatry because of the loss of the first-person perpective. The authors give some examples of individual accounts of experiences of depression which are only very partially covered by the *DSM*, among which those of William Styron and Andrew Solomon. The telling title of the section in question is: 'A new psychiatric syndrome?'

19 Kraepelin treads in the footsteps of his master Wilhelm Griesinger, whom Shorter considers to be the father of psychiatry. Griesinger's famous statement, 'All mental diseases are brain diseases', is mostly misunderstood, says Dillmann; it was explicitly meant to be a hypothesis. And because it is only a hypothesis, Griesinger wrote, we need to stick to the 'outside of the phenomena' (Dillmann 1990: 89ff). That is exactly what the *DSM*, from its third edition onwards, orders us to do.

20 Shorter speaks of 'a reembrace of the positivistic principles of the nineteenth century' (Shorter 1997: 302).

21 Shorter quotes one of the members of the *DSM-III* taskforce: '"When we started out with DSM, it was quite hard-nosed. If you didn't have data for a diagnosis, then screw it. Then Spitzer said if there's a group in favor, we'll take it." Somehow, neither the public nor the profession ever quite understood that this is what happened' (Shorter 2013: 133).

22 Cf Horwitz and Wakefield 2007: 212ff.

23 Cf Mayes and Horwitz 2005: 263: 'The DSM-III unintentionally positioned psychopharmacology on a growth trajectory that various institutions – insurance companies, managed care organizations, pharmaceutical companies and the government – propelled significantly in subsequent years as they responded to the *DSM-III*'s new diagnostic guidelines and the research incentives that it fostered.' Cf 255: 'The symptom-based diseases that the new manual would create greatly facilitated the expanding role of drug treatment in psychiatry. Psychoanalysis, in contrast, was becoming further marginalized because of its inability to respond to the growing need to treat seriously mentally ill persons in community settings and

to provide the specific disease entities that were required before a drug could be marketed and prescribed.' The talking cure made way for pharmacotherapy. This started with the development of benzodiazepines in 1950s, with Valium as peak. 'The benzodiazepines had a dramatic impact on the practice of psychiatry,' Shorter writes in his history book, making psychiatry more and more a discipline oriented on the supply of medication (Shorter 1997: 319).

24 Mayes and Horwitz (2005: 251) write: 'By the 1970s, the clients of dynamic psychiatrists were people with poor marriages, troubled children, failed ambitions, general nervousness, and diffuse anxiety … In addition, dynamic assumptions pervaded the treatment of deviant behavior in schools, juvenile courts, and child guidance clinics.'

25 There is a powerful European tradition, Shorter writes, of seeing depression inherently connected to anxiety. Cf Glas 2003. Cf Hartmut Rosa in *Resonanz* on the frequent absence of anxiety in the experience of depression (Rosa 2016: 202). Is Rosa following the experiences of the depressed there, or rather the symptomatographics of the *DSM*?

26 Though, for diplomatic reasons, in *DSM-III* the minor version of depression still had neurosis added in brackets, as if to emphasize what was being ruled out; this less severe depression was termed 'dysthymic disorder (neurotic depression)'. Besides that, there was the more severe subtype of melancholic depression, 'with melancholia', according to Shorter a pale shadow of historic melancholia and a useless category (Shorter 2013: 140).

27 Halfway through the book (111) Horwitz and Wakefield refer to the *DSM* definition of mental disorder, which states that the syndrome or pattern involved should 'be considered a manifestation of a behavioral, psychological, or biological dysfunction in the individual', on which they comment that the diagnostic criteria for the particular disorders have never been aligned with this general definition of mental disorder. This implies, they write, 'that the criteria for MDD [major depressive disorder] are invalid because they misclassify intense but naturally selected loss responses as disorder'.

28 Translated in 2009 as *The Weariness of the Self : Diagnosing the History of Depression in the Contemporary Age*.

29 Translated in 2013 as *Social Acceleration: A New Theory of Modernity*.

30 Translated in 2008 as *The Art of Shrinking Heads: On the New Servitude of the Liberated in the Age of Total Capitalism*.

31 The title, *The Perverse City*, refers to the Augustinian order of *De Civitate Dei*, which in the longlasting 'liberal cultural revolution' was gradually inverted, and so perverted.

32 This had a minor impact on the *DSM*. In *DSM-IV* (1994) an appendix entitled Outline for Cultural Formulation and Glossary of Culture-Bound Syndromes was added, part of which in *DSM-5* (2013) was promoted to the main text. Cultural psychiatry, however, one could say, is still largely 'appendix' instead of 'main text'.

33 See Kleinman and Good 1985: 'some psychobiological reality … that is being labeled differently in the two societies'; and: 'bodily complaints may metaphorically express personal and interpersonal distress' (438). Cf 247/256: 'concept of universal antecedents', related to 'distress responses'; and 282: 'the affect of depression' is universal, depression as 'illness' is not.

34 Term used by Obeyesekere in his chapter in *Culture and Depression* (147, cf 467), later title of a book he wrote on 'symbolic transformation in psychoanalysis and anthropology' (1990). The term refers to the word used by Freud for the restricting effect culture has on the drives – *Kulturarbeit* – for instance, in the following famous quote: 'Wo Es war, soll Ich werden./Es ist Kulturarbeit etwa wie der Trockenlegung der Zuydersee' (Freud 1976: 516). The meaning of 'work of culture' is different in this chapter: here it refers to culture-specific narratives and practices by and through which mental disorders are constituted and interpreted differently.

35 Cf Horwitz and Wakefield's criticism in *Loss of Sadness*. They speak of 'a confused postmodernist perspective that regards more or less everything human as thoroughly culturally determined' (2007: 195ff). It is the same kind of criticism as that of the well-known neo-Kraepelinian G.L. Klerman, in a review of *Culture and Depression* two years after its publication (Klerman 1987).

36 'Work of culture', Kleinman and Good 1985: 147, 467; depression as 'social affect' or 'drama' that is staged in a particular way in a particular sociocultural context, ibid.: 108, 188, 230, 429; 'transactional' nature of depression, ibid.: 113, 230 and especially 439, 493; 'somatization' versus 'psychologization', ibid.: 429ff.

37 Rosa himself, inspired among others by Fuchs, also comes to such a phenomenological move, by developing a sociological theory of 'resonance' in his magnum opus with the same title, *Resonanz* (2016). This work is the optimistic counterpart of the rather pessimistically ending *Beschleunigung* (2005). In the latter work Rosa was looking for an answer, in the former he might have found one: 'If acceleration is the problem, then resonance is possibly the solution,' so the book opens (13). Because of the fact that *Resonanz* was published while finishing this volume, I had to refrain from integrating it into this chapter.

38 Husserl's classical maxim 'To the matter itself', often referred to in phenomenological writings. The maxim summons us to bracket the 'natural disposition' and go back to the phenomenon as it is 'given', which means in the context of this chapter to get access to 'depression' as it is *experienced*, or, in other words, to open up a *concealed* level of experience in the thing today commonly termed '(major) depression'.

39 Hubertus Tellenbach, *Melancholie. Problemgeschichte, Endogenität, Typologie, Pathogenese, Klinik* (4th edition, 1983). *Depression in Japan* (2012), by medical anthropologist Junko Kitanaka, tells the story of the elimination of the traditional Japanese understanding of depressive states in terms of *ki* (life energy), after the invasion of German biopsychiatry in Japan around 1900. From *ki* to brain, so to speak. The irony of this story is that the concept of *Typus Melancholicus* – put forward by Tellenbach in the different editions of his famous work *Melancholie* (1961, 1974, 1976, 1983) – played a pivotal rol in the final succes of biopsychiatry in Japan. What happened in Japan via the concept of *Typus Melancholicus* is the exact opposite of what phenomenology aims at, which is, in this case, to get to the *experience* of depression. The present Japanese idiom of depression, Kitanaka writes, is 'curiously devoid of individual agency', psychiatric discourse 'falls short of becoming an internally persuasive, *experiential* language' (Kitanaka 2012: 13). Tellenbach, by the way, refers in *Melancholie* to the *ki*-notion, in the light of 'rhythmicity as basic vitality form' (Tellenbach 1983: 26).

40 See, for a related but different angle – that of 'affect theory' – for instance, recent work of German philosopher Jan Slaby (2016a, 2016b)

41 As said in note 35, Horwitz and Wakefield take Obeyesekere's position as an example of 'a confused postmodernist perspective' which considers almost everything human as deeply culturally defined. Again, they state that the 'philosophical depression' Obeyesekere speaks about involves normal sadness and not mental disorder; according to them the Singhalese anthropologist simply ignores the cases in which the sadness becomes pathological – that is, harmfully dysfunctional (Horwitz and Wakefield 2007: 195). But what they themselves ignore is the crucial point Obeyesekere makes here about the 'anchoring' of devastating hopelessness or despair.

42 The concept of alienation, which had been abondoned by critical theory, is reintroduced by Rosa in his *Soziologie der Weltbeziehung* ('sociology of world relation') by redefining it in a nonessentialist way as the opposite of 'resonance': 'the basic categories of *resonance* and *alienation* as the two complementary fundamental forms of world relation' (Rosa 2016: 72, see also Rosa 2010, 2012).

References

Acta Psychiatrica Scandinavica (2007): 115(s433), February: 4–183.

Alvarez, A. (2002/1971): *The Savage God: A Study of Suicide*. London: Bloombury.

APA (2013): *DSM-5. Diagnostic Manual of Mental Disorders*. Washington/London: American Psychiatric Association.

APA (2014): *DSM-5. Handboek voor de Classificatie van Psychische Stoornissen*. Amsterdam: Boom.

Bergh, B. van den (2013): Depression: resisting ultra-liberalism? In: Keohane, K. and Petersen, A. (eds), *The Social Pathologies of Contemporary Civilization*. Farnham: Ashgate.

Berrios, G.E. and Porter, R. (eds) (1995): *A History of Clinical Psychiatry: The Origin and History of Psychiatric Disorders*. London: Athlone Press.

Dillmann, R. (1990): *Alzheimer's Disease: The Concept of Disease and the Construction of Medical Knowledge*. Amsterdam: Thesis.

Dowrick, C. (2009): *Beyond Depression: A New Approach to Understanding and Management*, 2nd edn. Oxford/New York: Oxford University Press.

Dowrick, C. (2013): Depression as a culture-bound syndrome: implications for primary care. *British Journal of General Practice*, May: 229–30.

Dufour, D.-R. (2003): *L'Art de Réduire les Têtes. Sur la nouvelle servitude de l'homme libérale à l'ère du capitalisme total*. Paris: Éditions Denoël.

Dufour, D.-R. (2007): *Le Divin Marché. La Révolution Culturelle Libérale*. Paris: Éditions Denoël.

Dufour, D.-R. (2008): *The Art of Shrinking Heads: On the New Servitude of the Liberated in the Age of Total Capitalism*. Cambridge: Polity.

Dufour, D.-R. (2009): *La Cité Perverse. Libéralisme et Pornographie*. Paris: Éditions Denoël.

Dufour, D.-R. (2011): *L'Individu Qui Vient … Après le Libéralisme*. Paris: Éditions Denoël.

Dufour, D.-R. (2012): *Il Était une Fois le Dernier Homme*. Paris: Éditions Denoël.

Dufour, D.-R. (2014): *Le Délire Occidental*. Paris: Les Liens Qui Libèrent.

Dufour, D.-R. (2015): *Pléonexie*. Lormont: Le Bord de L'eau.

EDA (n.d.) *Depression Manifesto*. In: http://eddas.eu/our-manifesto (accessed 23 June 2016).

Ehrenberg, A. (1998): *La Fatigue d'Être Soi. Dépression et Société*. Paris: Éditions Odile Jacob.

Ehrenberg, A. (2010a): *La Société du Malaise*. Paris: Éditions Odile Jacob.

Ehrenberg, A. (2010b): *The Weariness of the Self. Diagnosing the History of Depression in the Contemporary Age*. Montreal and Kingston: McGill-Queen's University Press.

Freud, S. (1976): *Vorlesungen zur Einführung in die Psychoanalyse Und Neue Folge*. Frankfurt am Main: Fischer.

Fuchs, T. (2000): *Psychopathologie von Leib und Raum. Phänomenologisch-empirische Untersuchungen zu depressiven und paranoiden Erkrankungen*. Darmstadt: Steinkopff.

Fuchs, T. (2001): Melancholia as a desynchronization: towards a psychopathology of interpersonal time. *Psychopathology*, 34: 179–86.

Fuchs, T. (2002): The phenomenology of shame, guilt and the body in body dysmorphic disorder and depression. *Journal of Phenomenological Psychology*, 33: 223–43.

Fuchs, T. (2005): Corporealized and disembodied minds. A phenomenological view of the body in melancholia and schizophrenia. *Philosophy, Psychiatry and Psychology*, 12: 95–107.

Fuchs, T. (2010): Phenomenology and psychopathology. In: Gallagher, S. and Schmicking, D. (eds), *Handbook of Phenomenology and the Cognitive Sciences*. Dordrecht: Springer: 547–73.

Fuchs, T. (2011): Temporality and psychopathology. *Phenomenology and the Cognitive Sciences*. DOI 10.1007/s11097-010-9189-4.
Fuchs, T. (2013): Depression, intercoprorality and interaffectivity. *Journal of Consciousness Studies*, 20(7–8): 219–38.
Fuchs, Th. and Berger, M. (eds) (2013): *Affektive Störungen: Klinik – Therapie – Perspektiven*. Stuttgart: Schattauer.
Glas, G. (2003): A conceptual history of anxiety and depression. In: den Boer, J.A. and Sitsen, A. (eds), *Handbook on Anxiety and Depression*, 2nd edn. New York/Basel/Hong Kong: Marcel Dekker: 1–48.
Horwitz, A.V. and Wakefield, J.C. (2007): *The Loss of Sadness: How Psychiatry Transformed Normal Sorrow into Depressive Disorder*. Oxford/New York: Oxford University Press.
Ingenkamp, K. (2012): *Depression und Gesellschaft. Zur Erfindung einer Volkskrankheit*. Bielefeld: Transkript.
Jilek, W.G. (1995): Emil Kraepelin and comparative sociocultural psychiatry. *European Archives of Psychiatry and Clinical Neuroscience*, 245: 231–8.
Jilek, W.G. (2014): The early history of cultural psychiatry (1820–1980). *World Cultural Psychiatry Research Review*, 9(1): 3–15.
Keohane, K. and Petersen, A. (eds) (2013): *The Social Pathologies of Contemporary Civilization*. Farnham: Ashgate.
Kitanaka, J. (2012): *Depression in Japan: Psychiatric Cures for a Society in Distress*. Princeton, NJ/Oxford: Princeton University Press.
Kleinman, A. and Good, B. (eds) (1985): *Culture and Depression: Studies in the Anthropology and Cross-cultural Psychiatry of Affect and Disorder*. Berkeley: University of California Press.
Klerman, G.L. (1987): Book review of *Culture and Depression*. *Social Science and Medicine*, 24(9): 785–90.
Lee, S. (1999): Diagnosis postponed: shenjing shuairuo and the transformation of psychiatry in post-Mao China. *Culture, Medicine and Psychiatry*, 23: 349–80.
Mayes, R. and Horwitz, A.V. (2005): '*DSM-III* and the revolution in the classification of mental illness'. *Journal of the History of the Behavioral Sciences*, 41(3): 249–67.
Milders, F. and Thunissen, M. (2015): *Psychotherapeutische Psychiatrie. Menselijke Maat in Praktijk en Wetenschap*. Utrecht: De Tijdstroom.
Obeyesekere, G. (1990): *The Work of Culture*. Chicago: University of Chicago Press.
Ratcliffe, M. (2008): *Feelings of Being: Phenomenology, Psychiatry and the Sense of Reality*. Oxford: Oxford University Press.
Ratcliffe, M. (2015): *Experiences of Depression: A Study in Phenomenology*. Oxford: Oxford University Press.
Rosa, H. (2005): *Beschleunigung. Die Veränderung der Zeitstrukturen in der Moderne*. Frankfurt am Main: Suhrkamp.
Rosa, H. (2010): *Alienation and Acceleration: Towards a Critical Theory of Late-Modern Temporality*. Malmö: NSU Press.
Rosa, H. (2012): *Weltbeziehungen im Zeitalter der Beschleunigung. Umrisse einer neuen Gesellschaftskritik*. Berlin: Suhrkamp.
Rosa, H. (2013): *Social Acceleration: A New Theory of Modernity*. New York: Columbia University Press.
Rosa, H. (2016): *Resonanz. Eine Soziologie der Weltbeziehung*. Berlin: Suhrkamp.
Rosa, H. and Endres, W. (2016): *Resonanzpädagogik. Wenn es im Klassenzimmer knistert*. Wennheim/Basel: Belz.
Schotte, J. (1982): Comme dans la vie, en psychiatrie … Les perturbations de l'humeur comme troubles de base de l'éxistence. In: *Qu' est-ce que l'homme? Philosophie/*

psychanalyse. Hommage à Alphonse De Waelhens (1911–1981). Brussels: Publications des Facultés universitaires: 621–73.

Schotte, J. (1989): From redefining depressions to reassessing 'nosology' in present-day psychiatry: a three-fold post-script to the papers of van Praag and van den Hoofdakker. In: *Biological Psychiatry: Marching Backwards into the Future*. Leuven: Leuven University Press: 61–110.

Schuster, D. (2011): *Neurosthenic Nation: America's Search for Health, Happiness and Comfort*. New Brunswick: Rutgers University Press.

Shorter, E. (1997): *A History of Psychiatry: From the Era of the Asylum to the Age of Prozac*. New York: John Wiley and Sons.

Shorter, E. (2013): *How Everyone Became Depressed: The Rise and Fall of the Nervous Breakdown*. Oxford: Oxford University Press.

Shorter, E. and Fink, M. (2010): *Endocrine Psychiatry: Solving the Riddle of Melancholia*. Oxford: Oxford University Press.

Slaby, J. (2016a): Relational affect. Working Paper SFB 1171 Affective Societies 02/16.

Slaby, J. (2016b): Affektive Relationalität. In: Eberlein, U. (ed.), *Zwischenleiblichkeit und bewegtes Verstehen – Intercorporeity, Movement and Tacit Knowledge*. Bielefeld: Transcript.

Solomon, A. (2002): *The Noonday Demon: An Anatomy of Depression*. London: Vintage.

Tellenbach, H. (1983): *Melancholie. Problemgeschichte, Endogenität, Typologie, Pathogenese, Klinik*. Berlin: Springer.

Tseng, W.-S., Jilek, W, Bartocci, G. and Bhui K. (2014): The recent history of cultural psychiatry (1971–2012). *World Cultural Psychiatry Research Review*, 9(1): 16–25.

5 Alzheimer's disease

A social pathology of contemporary civilization

Kieran Keohane

This chapter explores the sociological grounds of Alzheimer's disease and the amnesia and cognitive decline that are purported to be its symptoms in terms of the collective existential conditions associated with mutations of the symbolic order and institutional structure of the contemporary age. Alzheimer's disease, like 'anxiety' and 'depression', is an elastic and vague individualist biomedical-neuropathological diagnostic category, a disease diagnosed always by inference, that can be confirmed only on autopsy, by the presence of 'amyloid plaques' and 'tau tangles' in brain tissue, about which there is a great deal of uncertainty. The presence or absence of biomarkers of Alzheimer's tells us very little about dementia, which may have many other causes ranging from deformations of the brain related to aging, to cerebral ischemia due to arterio-sclerosis, to stroke and to brain injury, to co-morbidity with Parkinson's disease, multiple sclerosis (MS) and numerous other chronic conditions, to alcohol and substance abuse and so on, so much so that, in the face of 'the enigma of the brain' (Blum 2012), 'Alzheimer's disease' becomes a generic catch-all for dementia, not only as a common-sense understanding among the general public but for the medical profession too. In fact, the standard medical position on the status of Alzheimer's disease in particular in relation to the concept of dementia in general is, as represented in this instance by the *Oxford Textbook of Old Age Psychiatry*, which states baldly: 'Despite billions of dollars being spent on the condition over the past several decades, there are no diagnostic tests or even neuropathological changes that can precisely define the difference between someone who's brain is aging and someone who has Alzheimer's' (Denning and Thomas 2013: 372).[1]

The Nun Study: brain reserve or quality of vocation?

The most famous epidemiological study of Alzheimer's disease is the so-called Nun Study. Very briefly, the Nun Study is an ongoing longitudinal epidemiological study, commenced in 1986, initiated by David Snowdon at the University of Kentucky Medical School, and since 2009 at the University of Minnesota. It involves 678 nuns of the School Sisters of Notre Dame from convents in the American mid-west who have agreed to undertake regular psychometric testing and to donate their brains post-mortem for autopsy. The Nun Study has so far generated numerous research publications in leading international medical and scientific journals including the *Lancet*, the *Journal of the American Medical Association*, journals in neurology, gerontology and epidemiology, as well as in the general media – *Time* and the *New York Times*, for instance.

The essential summary text is Snowdon's (2001) *Aging With Grace: What the Nun Study Teaches us about Leading Longer, Healthier and More Meaningful Lives.*[2] In Snowdon's title our concern with Alzheimer's and the dementia reputed to it is articulated with the idea of life as being 'meaningful'. We note also the use of the word 'grace', by which Snowdon seems to acknowledge and respect the particularity of the women in his study; that these elderly women are nuns, and that the idea of 'grace' [*charis*/charisma] – the Divine gift of their vocation, their 'calling' – is an important source of meaningfulness in their lives.[3]

> Prayer and worship are at the core of the sisters' lives at every age and stage of health. While we cannot directly measure intangibles such as faith and social support, the Nun Study would be incomplete without acknowledging their powerful influence.
>
> Ibid.: 116–17

Because 'faith and social support' are 'intangible and cannot be directly measured' Snowdon has no means of handling them. Analysing their 'powerful influence' is the task that we take up here, which we will begin by disarticulating 'faith' and 'social support', formulating faith in terms of vocation/calling/*Beruf* and social support in terms of how the nuns' lives are embedded in the symbolic order and imaginative structures of the convent. To begin we take note also of the word 'leading' in Snowdon's title. Human beings do not simply 'live' their lives in the same way that other biological organisms live; as human beings we *lead* our lives; that is to say, human life is oriented towards something more than biological imperatives of survival and reproduction; human life is life that is *led*; led by the light of ideals; and human life is life that *follows*: life that follows causes and callings emanating from transcendental sources of authority. This is the source of the meaningfulness of human life.[4]

To get a sense of the importance of what is passed over in silence in the Nun Study let us hear Max Weber on how leading one's life in answer to a strong vocation structures mind in service to an idea; and it is significant that Weber is speaking of 'science as a vocation', though he speaks also of the vocation of the artist (and he alludes to the vocation of the entrepreneur and the military leader), for – while they each appear to be different – 'the psychological qualities do not differ. Both are frenzy (in the sense of Plato's "mania") and inspiration' (Weber 1968/1919: 296). Weber makes a distinction between working scientists and the scientist who is capable of coming up with a genuinely new idea, and that difference, Weber says, depends on the quality of the scientist's vocation. Science requires not only 'cool intellect ... [and] a firm and reliable work procedure … but one's very "heart and soul", for Nothing is worthy of man as man unless he can pursue it with passionate devotion' (ibid.: 295). In his other famous essay on 'Politics as a Vocation', Weber (1978/1919: 223) talks about the person who is 'conscious that his life has a *meaning* in the service of a "cause"' [emphasis in the original]; a person who becomes 'aware of a responsibility for the consequences of his conduct and really feels such responsibility with heart and soul' (ibid.: 225). And in *The Protestant Ethic and the Spirit of Capitalism*, on the theme of Luther's conception of the 'calling' – *Beruf*[5] – vocation – even though in this context Weber is discussing the meaning of vocation in the Protestant church, it applies here to these Catholic nuns in a teaching order, for a vocation is 'a religious conception, a task set by God … a life task, a definite field in which to work' (1976/1905: 79). Weber's formulation of the fundamental importance of *Beruf* to the meaning of life has strong affinity with Antonovsky's paradigm of salutogenesis – how a 'sense of coherence', 'a global orientation that expresses the extent to which one has a pervasive, enduring though dynamic feeling of confidence in the comprehensibility, manageability and above all the meaningfulness' of one's being in the world plays a vital role in health and longevity (Antonovsky 1987: 19).

We can imagine, Weber says, a scientist who 'may be an excellent worker and yet never have had any valuable idea of his own' (1968/1919: 295). Similarly we can imagine that there are Sisters who are excellent nuns and yet the quality of their vocation is less intense, lacking what Plato identifies as the decisive 'mania', the passionate devotion, enthusiasm and inspiration that may characterize the vocations of other Sisters. My hypothesis is that it is the quality of vocation that keeps the mind clearly focused on radiant ideals that affords some of the Sisters in the Nun Study more protection from dementia. And generalizing this hypothesis from the particular case of the Nun Study, my argument will be that the erosion of the possibility of coherently pursuing a meaningful vocation under conditions of post-modernism, neoliberalism and social acceleration, namely transformations of the symbolic order and of the moral foundations of economy and society, are the sociological sources of dementia as symptomatic of the social pathologies of contemporary civilization – not so much as the normal senility of an aged civilization but rather as a metastasis of malignant developments[6] that corrode the foundations of consciousness.

To examine this hypothesis, we focus on the essential findings of the Nun Study concerning 'grammatical complexity' and 'idea density' and the related hypothesis of 'brain reserve'. Briefly, the nuns, on entering the convent, had been required to write an autobiographical essay on their family background and social circumstances, reflecting on their reasons and feelings on taking up convent life. When these essays were analysed some 50, 60, even 70 years after they had been written, Snowdon and his colleague, psycholinguist Susan Kemper, found an extraordinarily strong positive correlation between the grammatical complexity and the idea density of those early essays and the nuns' later protection from Alzheimer's (Snowdon 2001: 112).

'Grammatical complexity' measures in a range from simple one-clause sentences to complex sentences with multiple forms of embedding and subordination; the articulacy of one's linguistic structure is related to cognitive functioning as working memory. 'Idea density' measures the number of individual ideas expressed per ten words, and thus is related to such psycholinguistic qualities as vocabulary and loquaciousness, succinctness, clarity and precision in grasping and expressing ideas, and also in the use of simile, allegory and metaphor to suggest and to infer more ideas than are actually made explicit. Thus, idea density is related to higher order cognitive faculties and qualities of mind, such as abstract thinking, synthesis of ideas, and imagination. The essential finding of the Nun Study is that the more grammatical complexity and idea density contained in an essay written by a nun in her late teens, the more likely that nun would be Alzheimer's free in her 80s and 90s. Snowdon and his team interpret grammatical complexity and idea density as indices of individual intelligence and education, hypothesizing that the more intelligent nuns, especially if they had continued their education throughout the life course, developed more 'brain reserve', and this brain reserve insulates them against the effects of brain atrophy, neuro-degeneration, plaques and tangles, things that can be measured, by brain imaging and, on autopsy, by brain weight, morphology and histopathology. The brain reserve [or cognitive reserve] hypothesis has subsequently become a standard and central idea in neuropsychiatric and psychological understandings of Alzheimer's disease and the dementia reputed to it (Fratiglioni and Hui-Xin: 2007).

But rather than treating grammatical complexity and idea density as indices of an individual-psychological quantity of brain reserve, we might rather see such complexity and density as indices of sociological and existential *quality*: indices of variations in the richness (or otherwise) of the meaning-bearing symbolic order and imaginaries within which the nuns live their lives. So to see what is really going on in 'brain reserve', let us re-examine some data from the research:

> I was born September 26th, 1909, the eldest of seven children, five girls and two boys.... [M]y candidate year was spent in the Motherhouse teaching Chemistry and Second Year Latin at Notre Dame Institute. With God's grace I intend to do my best for our Order, for the spread of Religion, and for my personal sanctification.
>
> Cited by Kemper *et al.* 2001, in Ingram 2014: 120

By contrast:

> God started my life off well by bestowing up me a grace of inestimable value.... The past year which I have spent as a candidate studying at Notre Dame College has been a very happy one. Now I look forward with eager joy to receiving the Holy Habit of Our Lady and to a life of union with Love Divine.
>
> Ibid.

The first statement (from a nun who developed dementia) is articulate, factual and goal-oriented. She herself is at the centre of the narrative: 'I was born September 26th' … etc., and one might even say it is egoistically instrumental, in terms of her expressed self-interest in 'my personal sanctification'. The second passage (from a nun who did not develop dementia) is quite different, but the striking difference is not so much in terms of quantity of grammatical complexity and idea density, but rather of a qualitative difference: the role of a big Other – God, the Name of the Father – in leading the narrative – 'God started my life off well …' and the 'passionate devotion and enthusiasm' she expresses in answering her vocation.

Listen again for the difference between Sister Helen and Sister Emma:

> I was born at Eau Claire, Wis., on May 24th 1913, and was baptized in St James' Church. My Father, Mr L.M. Hallacher was born in the city of Ross, Co. Cork, Ireland, and is now a sheet metal worker in Eau Claire. There are ten children in the family, six boys and four girls. Two of the boys are dead.
>
> Sister Helen, who developed dementia. Snowdon 2001: 110

> Already two, a brother and a sister, had begun the family which would gradually reach the number eight.… When I was in the fourth grade death visited our family taking one to whom I was particularly attached, my little brother Karl, who was but a year and a half old. He was called to his 'Home' after three weeks of very much suffering on Good Friday early in the morning. The pastor was willing to have the funeral services before Easter, but I was hoping and praying that my parents would not consent, for I thought, since he died on Good Friday he might be in our midst, living, on Easter Sunday. The services were held on Monday morning, which I was privileged to attend since we were quarantined.
>
> Sister Emma, who did not develop dementia. Ibid.: 111

There is no doubt that the second is not only much more grammatically complex, and also that there is far greater idea density, but while these two empirically measurable quantifiable indices are clearly obvious, such quantification misses the essential difference – which concerns the quality of vocation. The first recounts and enumerates banal realities of ordinary life, whereas the second tells us of a really quite extraordinary experience: the death of her brother on the most auspicious day of the Christian calendar, Good Friday, the day of Christ's passion and crucifixion; the answering of Sister Emma's fervent hopes and prayers, in one sense, that her brother's funeral would be postponed until Monday in the hope that her brother may be resurrected on Easter Sunday. He wasn't resurrected, of course, and one might expect that Emma would have taken this experience of grief and suffering, hope and then bitter disappointment as refuting her faith, but somehow it has had the opposite effect.

In this vignette Sister Emma isn't simply recounting some ordinary event in her family biography, nor is she telling us the sad, bald fact of her brother's death, as Sister Helen does. Sister Emma is giving voice to the transfiguring power of her personal experience of epiphany, the moment when she feels that God revealed Himself and showed His divine power to her. God seemed to answer Emma's prayers, but at the same time He left her important prayer unanswered. Whatever science may make of this as intangible, unquantifiable and, thereby, irrelevant; whatever reasonable, secular people may make of this doesn't matter one iota here. What really matters is that a ten-year-old girl who would become Sister Emma had what she understands to have been a miraculous experience. Emma was transfigured by her experience; it stamped her indelibly; it affected her profoundly; it transfixed her. The subject 'Sister Emma' was formed at that moment, by her experiencing herself as being subject to the absolute power of a big Other. To Emma's mind, God manifested Himself to her; He partially answered her prayers, but at the same time He left her most passionate desire thwarted and denied, and thereby perpetually renewed as it circles around the trauma and becomes Sister Emma's fixation. God calls for more than a child's prayer; Sister Emma is transfixed in *béance*; she must answer her calling. Sister Emma is one of the nuns 'with the words', not because perhaps 'her mother read more to her when she was a child' or some such mundane quantifiable influence (ibid.: 117), but because she believes that she has been given *charisma*, the gift of the Holy Spirit, the gift of tongues with which to proclaim the Good News.

We will take one more example, to elaborate the 'quality of vocation' hypothesis further. The case is that of the parallel beginnings and the sharply diverging endings of Sister Maria and Sister Dolores, two young Bavarian Novices who emigrated from Nazi Germany to America on the same boat in 1937. Sister Maria died aged 83, having suffered dementia for several years; previously, due to several bouts of ill health and two nervous breakdowns, she had withdrawn from teaching to work in the tapestry room. In stark contrast, Sister Dolores had a full and successful teaching career, completing Masters and Doctoral degrees in her 50s; at the age of 70 she fulfilled what she says had always been her life-long dream, when she sought and took up a post in Kenya as a missionary, where she led a large development project. After ten years Sister Dolores returned to America, still as sharp as a tack in her 80s, and scored a near perfect result in the Nun Study psychometric tests (ibid.: 68–79, *passim*).

A brief examination of their respective autobiographies reveals differences that will prove to be decisive. Sister Maria's early life is marked by difficulties. Her twin sister dies at birth, and she seems to bear some guilt for this as she recalls her mother saying that her childhood rambunctiousness had 'taken too much life from her twin'. During her teens Maria had to care for her father and her mother who both fell ill, became incapacitated and died. 'Maria was an orphan when she boarded the *Deutschland* and stepped into the unknown,' Snowdon says. '"What gave you the courage to leave?" I once asked her. She replied, "I knew God would provide all that I needed in America"' (ibid.: 68). What emerges clearly in this autobiographical vignette is that Sister Maria's vocation is characterized by flight from grief and insecurity due to the loss and dissolution of her parental household. Sister Maria is not so much answering a calling as she is being driven by necessity and by the hope that she would find a new big Other, God in America.

Sister Dolores's vocation is much more clearly a *Beruf*. Her life course is a career; the fulfilment of a God-given task in a definite field; her life is charged with meaningfulness and sense of coherence as she pursues a cause and it leads her towards realizing an ideal through dedicated hard work. In her autobiography Sister Dolores recalls her first experience with the School Sisters of Notre Dame when she attended their school, which she loved. 'She came home from school one day and announced to her parents: "I love school, I love learning, and I love Jesus. I want to be a priest". She wanted to be a Jesuit, free to spend the rest of her life immersed in both intellectual and spiritual pursuits' (ibid.: 71, *passim*). Dolores has not just one, but two powerful vocations, professional and religious; and then comes the moment when the two vocations, belonging to temporal and sacred realms respectively, become synthesized and fused into one. Dolores was working as assistant principal at a public school run by the School Sisters of Notre Dame when, in 1937, an official letter arrived instructing all teachers to drop their affiliations to religious congregations and to join the Nazi party. The instruction from a third party, the command from the *Führer*, with its dubious claim to authority, has the unintended consequence of being the agent of forging Dolores's other two as-yet uncertain vocations into one. The letter is the catalyst for Dolores's transfiguring and transfixing conversion experience: '"Anger, frustration and fear shook my very being," she says. Walking back towards the convent, "my mind cleared and my heart vowed", and within two weeks Dolores had entered the convent as a novice' (ibid.: 72, *passim*). Temporal and sacred realms are reconciled and synthesized into a new overarching, transcendental and unified symbolic order, a big Other with absolute authority. Authorized by that big Other, Dolores's life course becomes an exemplary demonstration of what constitutes a true vocation: 'enthusiasm and hard work, and above all both of them jointly' (Weber 1968/1919: 295) expended in the pursuit of a cause, in fulfilment of a life task set by God in a definite field of work. Dolores does not suffer dementia partly since she is answering a powerful, resonant, meaningful vocation on a royal road brightly illuminated by the radiant ideals on which she has her mind set.

The imaginative structure of a nun's life: social support in a total institution

Just as an intangible like 'faith' can be formulated, analysed and empirically measured in terms of quality of vocation, we turn now to an analysis of the powerful influence of 'social support', which we can make tangible and empirically analyse by formulating it in terms of the imaginative structure of a nun's life as it is embedded and cultivated within the convent. Our argument here is that a nun's protection from the dementia reputed to Alzheimer's disease is an effect not only of the quality of her vocation on entry, but also of the integrity and consistency of her vocation over the course of her lifespan; and that this consistency and sense of coherence is due to 'social support' in the form of the symbolic order and imaginative structure of convent life as 'a mosaic of interpretive courses of action, an ensemble of practices of engagement and orientations' (Blum 2003: 31) forming the nuns' day-to-day consciousness and self-awareness.

The nuns' lives are entirely ruled by the Name of the Father. The nuns take solemn vows, of poverty, chastity and obedience. They live under the Holy Rule; they are subject to 'Holy Orders' from the most transcendental of authorities – God Himself. As 'brides of Christ' they are *Hausfrauen* of an ideal husband, and their lives are devoted to the mindful care and maintenance of an immaculately orderly household. And, underneath that sacred symbolic order, the imaginative structure of their lives is organized within the convent as a 'total institution' (Goffman 1961),[7] a panoptical apparatus by means of which the powerful, penetrating, diffuse and omnipresent disciplinary gaze of a big Other is internalized and deeply subjectivized (Foucault 1991).

The nuns' thoughts, words and deeds, their innermost recesses of wish and will are structured and ordered. These nuns, from childhood (as reported prominently in their autobiographical recollections of the experiences that they say awakened their vocations – the sacramental rites of First Holy Communion, Confirmation etc.), all the way up through their lives as nuns, from the rituals of induction into the convent, through numerous rituals of mortification as well as spiritual transformation in their passage through clearly defined stages – Aspirancy, Postulancy, Novitiate, First Profession, Solemn Profession and so on – which are all formal *rites de passage* of incremental status elevation (Turner 1967); these are structuring and meaning-giving 'stamping experiences' for the Sisters individually as well as members of a cohort, for one of the functions of a *rite de passage* is to forge a spirit of *communitas* and solidarity among those who go through the experience together. As well as these major *rites de passage*, the nuns' each and every day is structured, governed and limited in accordance with a timetable – rising early, prayer, breakfast, work, lunch, mass, etc., even the short periods allocated to recreation are carefully structured. The nuns' lives are ordered and their minds are framed so as to ensure that there are no experiences of liminality and anti-structure. And, more precisely, moments wherein uncertainty may arise are themselves occasions that are explicitly built into formal *rites de passage*, overseen and managed by expert masters [or mistresses] of ceremonies and in accordance with deep traditions; so that, should a Sister have a personal crisis of faith, her moment of uncertainty is confessed, contemplated and folded back into her spiritual life in terms of it having been a trial sent by God and thus a necessary and meaningful suffering, thereby not only reducing the experience of liminality and anti-structure but moreover of using it to fortify structure.

For a prophylactic against the dementia reputed to Alzheimer's disease, here is the prescription that may be derived from the Nun Study: against the bewildering complexity of contemporary life, the nuns have simplicity; against the uncertainty and precarity of economic life, the nuns have security and permanency; against the experience of social acceleration the nuns live in an oasis of decelerated time; against a proliferating 'tyranny of choices' (Salecl 2011) the nuns have strictly limited choices; against decomposition of identity into a multiplicity of subject positions, the nuns have one identity (or no subjectivity – 'none'); against the socio-pathogenic incoherencies of contemporary civilization the nuns have sense of coherence and salutogenesis; against the dissolution of phallic signifiers into floating signifiers and asymbolia, the nuns have the Name of the Father; against the loss of meaningful metanarratives the nuns are heroines in 'the greatest story ever told'; against existential absurdity and the random thrownness of existence, the nuns have profound spiritual resonance with an eternal and absolute Truth.

Dementia as a social pathology of contemporary civilization: transformations of the symbolic order and the moral foundations of economy and society

The Nun Study teaches us two things about Alzheimer's disease: first, the importance of *Beruf* – vocation – pursuing a life task in a definite field of work in response to a calling from a big Other as a source of meaningfulness; and, second, the importance of being embedded in an institutional order and imaginative structure within which a vocation is supported and enabled to be coherently pursued. But the nuns belong to a pre-modern form of life in which the symbolic order and the moral foundations of economy and society are entirely different from those that underpin contemporary civilization.

The moral foundation of pre-modern society is 'mechanical solidarity': people are integrated on the principle of their similarity to one another. Correspondingly, in pre-modern society the symbolic order, the *conscience collective*,[8] is clear, coherent and all encompassing, and the source of meaning is a transcendent divinity, an omnipresent big Other as an absolute authority (Durkheim 1997/1893). These features of common life and of group mind are diametrically opposite to the individualized forms of life and of mind that characterize modern society, wherein the moral foundation is 'organic solidarity' – people's interdependence on the basis of their individual differences in the division of labour – and whereby the symbolic order – the *conscience collective*, the authority of the big Other – is multiple and differentiated. So we must leave behind the world of the convent, though we take with us the lessons that the nuns have taught us, and we look now at the ways in which accelerating transformations of the moral foundations and of the symbolic orders in modern, late and post-modern economy and society impact upon the conditions of possibility of having a vocation and of coherently pursuing it if we are to understand the sources of Alzheimer's disease as a social pathology of contemporary civilization.

Here I want to use the term 'contemporary' in two senses: first, in the sense of 'modern western civilization', conventionally understood as encompassing the early decades of the nineteenth to the late twentieth centuries;[9] and I will also use 'contemporary' in the more specific sense of the present and the recent past and emerging social forms and relationships, for Alzheimer's disease and the amnesia and cognitive decline that are taken to be its symptoms is not just a characteristic disease of modern western civilization, but the current 'epidemic' of Alzheimer's disease coincides with the two recent paradigmatic transformations of contemporary society, namely, the conditions of post-modernity and the neoliberal revolution, both of which begin in the 1970s and 1980s and both of which have entailed the continuity and also the amplification of pathogenic tendencies in modern civilization – and are also new mutations in their own right. Furthermore, as Rosa (2013) argues, these recent paradigmatic transformations – post-modernism and neoliberalism – are also to be understood as emerging from and contributing to the social acceleration that is an essential characteristic of the overarching history of modernity. The central thesis of Rosa's 'new theory of modernity' is of accelerated temporalization due to the recursive effects of technology-led acceleration (from the railway, through industrial manufacture, through flight, to the virtual instantaneity of digital technologies); the acceleration of social change (of social structures and institutions, of economy, politics and culture); and acceleration of the pace of life. These three dimensions of acceleration, recursively amplifying one another, have profound effects on subjective experience and identity, among which, and relevant to our discussion here, are pathologies of desynchronization and disintegration, whereby people are prone to find themselves 'out of step', 'out of joint', 'out of tune', or 'out of rhythm', as it were, with meaning-bearing social relations within social structures and institutions that are changing more and more quickly; and while dysrhythmia and dissonance may be generalized experiences for everyone living in societies with accelerating temporalization, the pathogenic effects may especially affect older people.

Desymbolization and anomie

Post-modernism means, among other things, the loss of faith in metanarratives and the consequent relativization of values (Lyotard 1984); the waning of historicity, a collective generalized forgetting about the past and a sense of living in a permanent present; intensifications and elaborations of individuality and identity and amplified emphasis on subjectivity and the self so that 'feelings' eclipse 'meanings' (Jameson 1991). Neoliberalism, among other things, entails the deregulation of economic relations in general and the flexibilization of work in particular, and thus the end of stable, life-long vocational careers and the 'corrosion of character', even for the professional classes, and insecurity – indeed, the precarity of working life more generally (Sennett 1998; Bourdieu 1999; Harvey 2007); privatization, and the complete penetration of the commodity form into all social relations; and an inverse trans-valuation of all values into market value. In Dufour's (2008) formulation, taken all together, the conditions of post-modernism and neoliberalism entail a pervasive process of desymbolization and thus a generalized *asymbolia*. This has profound ramifications for subject-formation, reaching even to the level of anthropological mutation, Dufour says, because the subject is formed within the symbolic order, through being subject to the Name of the Father. 'Man is, prior to his birth and beyond his death, caught up in the symbolic chain.... [T]he subject is the slave of discourse' (Lacan, in Dufour 2008: 155). Neoliberalism's cultural revolution is to disarticulate the symbolic chain, to dissolve its *points de capition*, to undermine and erase the ideals, the authorities, the values and traditions, the Name(s) of the Father that have formed modern subjects and 'in the name of' which individuals subordinate desires and direct their actions.

And as every revolution seeks to set afoot a new man, with the decomposition of the symbolic order comes a corresponding anthropological mutation: the emergence and cultivation of a new kind of subject. The subject of the neoliberal revolution, Dufour says, is uncritical (because historical bases and transcendental ideals that authorize critique have been undermined and relativized); hyper-individuated (because of flexibilization and new declensions in the division of labour); and amoral (because they are 'freed' from traditions and normative conventions as all relations become market relations and thus morally neutral).[10] The emerging neoliberal subject, Dufour (2011) says, is a Sadean isolist with psychotic tendencies.

Alzheimer's disease and the dementia reputed to it is a social pathology associated with conditions of post-modernism, neoliberalism and late modernity – the accelerating decomposition of traditional institutions and social roles; the ever more fine-grained differentiations, fragmentations and out-sourcings in the division of labour; ever more nuanced and ever more rapidly changing elaborations of individualism, identitarianism and the privatization of morality and so on – all of which we should acknowledge could appear as refinements of civilization in Durkheim's paradigm, so much so that, as with *Suicide*, Durkheim (2002/1897: 334) may say that the dementia associated with Alzheimer's disease is the price – 'the ransom money' – that we pay for modernity as a form of life.[11] Here we remind ourselves that Durkheim located the source of the suicidogenic currents that flowed and pulsed and swirled through modern European societies with older and deeper sea-changes of the moral foundations and symbolic orders of European civilization that were the Enlightenment, and before that the Reformation and the Renaissance, and with those changes a progressive loosening of the hold of the *conscience collective* over the individual and the emergence of the modern subject. In the late twentieth and early twenty-first centuries we have an equivalent sea-change, in the form of post-modernism, neoliberalism and accelerating temporalization, and it is precisely in coincidence with these more recent broad changes in western civilization that we can identify what we may call *dementiagenic* currents and find Alzheimer's disease becoming epidemic.

Durkheim shows how, in pre-modern societies, the individual subject, as we understand that term to mean today, scarcely existed at all. Instead, we find predominantly a 'group mind' – the *conscience collective*. Religion pervades the whole of life, constituting an entire world of common beliefs and practices that are held intensely by all members of the group, wherein authority is absolute. By contrast, in modern society the individual consciousness comes to the fore, and religion is only one domain among many differentiated spheres of life and activity, each one with its own autonomy and circumscribed authority. The source of this all-encompassing transformation from pre-modern to modern forms of life is the division of labour. Pre-modern society is integrated by mechanical solidarity and occupational similarity, so much so that 'the individual is submerged in the group' (Durkheim 1997/1893: 141–2); the subject is one with the collective as an integral whole; there is one Subject (Dufour 2008). Modern society entails a transformation of the moral foundation of society by 'the progressive preponderance of organic solidarity' (Durkheim 1997/1893: 126) and occupational specialization in the division of labour. Now, 'the group is eclipsed' (ibid.: 136) by 'the cult of the individual' (ibid.: 333) and individuality is expressed and demonstrated by one's unique and particular *Beruf*, in the economic sphere primarily, as 'occupation', and extending into other differentiated spheres of action and value with their own distinctive normative orders, so that the modern individual may have become several subjects, differentiated, though stabilized and mutually interdependent and capable of being encompassed within coherent sociological and biographical overarching narratives. Under conditions of post-modernity and neoliberalism, the conditions of possibility of constituting a subject through pursuing a *Beruf* are eroded and 'flexibilized' so much so that subjectivity becomes undermined and precarious, while at the same time it is accelerating and fragmenting into a multitude of proliferating, fleeting subject positions, isolations that cannot be encompassed into any coherent and meaningful narratives. Thus, post-modernism and neoliberalism are forms of life that, while they may appear as thriving growth, extensions and expansions in every which way, are, in fact, malignant and metastatic pathologies of contemporary civilization, among whose most characteristic symptoms is the corrosion of consciousness.

Herein lies the root of the social pathologies inherent in this great transformation of the moral foundations and the symbolic orders of contemporary civilization that Durkheim analysed in *Suicide*, foremost among them being *egoisme* and *anomie* (tendencies that are now reaching conditions of Sadean *isolism* in Dufour's account): egoism arising from the detachment of the individual from networks of social relations and institutions, and anomie from the dissolution of the *conscience collective*, the big Other as a source of singular authority. Durkheim's key concept, anomie, is derived from Greek, *anomia*, meaning 'no law'; more specifically the etymology is from the proto-Indo-European *nomn*, from whence '*nom*', 'noun', 'name'. *Anomie* means that there are no Name(s) of the Father, no phallic signifiers, no *points de capition* that fix the flow of signification in the social fabric and give order to the symbolic order. Where there are no big Other(s), there can be no metanarratives and there can be no memories – for memorable and meaningful experiences become memorable and meaningful only insofar as they are authorized or prohibited by the Father – hence they *matter.* Otherwise, they merely flit by, as ephemera and sensations. Without collective representations that function as phallic signifiers there can only be 'floating signifiers', shifting, sliding, relativized meanings, a decomposing *conscience collective*, a disintegrating social mind, leaving the weakened individual consciousness adrift. This is *de-mentia*, which means 'the leaving of mind': the gradual disintegration of individual consciousness from the *conscience collective*, and the *conscience collective* becoming unfixed, disordered and incoherent.

Loss of sources of the self

Desymbolization, undermining and weakening of the phallic signifiers that constitute the big Other means that there are no strong and transcendental collective representations, ideas to which the subject is subject, against which the subject can reflexively define him/herself, either in conformity with or in contradistinction to; no radiant ideals or authoritative sources of vocation. Thus, just as people are faced with the imperative of constituting themselves as subjects, they find that they are deprived of the symbolic resources that would make that project possible.

Within the broader context of modernity as *A Secular Age* (Taylor 2007) and the transformation of the *conscience collective*, modern subjectivity – with its imperative of individual self-creation and 'ethics of authenticity' – is now confronted with a loss of the 'sources of the self' (Taylor 1989) that had heretofore secured identity. 'A vision of the good becomes available for the people of a given culture through being given expression in some manner,' Taylor says (ibid.: 91). Moral and spiritual sources may be divine, or in the world, or in the powers of the self. In contemporary civilization the vision of the good is given expression through the division of labour, and thus in a person's finding within themselves, drawing out and cultivating their own authentic *Beruf*. For the modern subject the sources of the self are no longer given by a transcendental divinity, nor are they pre-assigned by the place of one's birth in the social order of the group; instead they are internal to the individual: sources of the modern self spring 'from the divinity that stirs within' (ibid.: 302). The prime motive of modern action becomes the individual's quest for authentic self-realization: the person must seek within themselves their unique attributes and aptitudes, bring forth, cultivate and develop them so that they become manifest in a life project; and the mode of action in which all of this takes place is in the domain of work – that is, in one's vocational career. The moral imperative has become identical with the economic imperative: dedication to one's authentic vocation, manifested by 'making a successful career for oneself', has become the secular equivalent of the fulfilment of 'a life task set by God'. Work becomes central to life as a transcendental experience (Dejours and Deranty 2010).

Once upon a time, Taylor says, those things that 'are part of the tacit background to objects of reliance, of things that are "ready to hand" in Heidegger's language' included the sincere belief and taken-for-grantedness of God's benevolent omnipresence. This is the case for some of the Sisters in the Nun

Study, but while it is undoubtedly the source of the serenity that characterizes the calm, clear minds of some of the elderly nuns as they approach the end of their lives (which for them is a new beginning in a higher life), from the point of view of late modernity theirs is an entirely exotic form of life, a residual trace persisting now as an 'island that time forgot' on the ocean of liquid modernity. As Taylor says, the theistic worldview has been shattered by modernity, and now 'virtually nothing in the domain of mythology, metaphysics, or theology stands in this fashion as publicly available background today' (1989: 491). Reading the general thesis of increasing individuation in the accelerating transition from tradition to modernity through the lens of Taylor's analysis of the amplifying imperative of authentic self-actualization while 'sources of the self' become transformed, from pre-determining to self-determining sources, Rosa, echoing Durkheim, argues that:

> in traditional societies (and well into early modernity) the substantial social identity of subjects was, as it were, fixed and predefined externally … tradition and religion show the premodern subject his/her place in the world and in society and predefine who it is, where it stands and what it has to do.
>
> Rosa 2013: 227

This has changed utterly. 'The development leading to modernity is a process of the *temporalization of life* … in which the course of a lifetime is a central structural principle; a form of life mainly ordered biographically' (ibid.: 246, emphasis in the original). And, as we have seen, for a biography to be coherent and meaningful it must be the story of a life that leads somewhere; a life that 'amounts to something' because it is a life that follows a *Beruf* in pursuit of some higher causes and ideals. But desymbolization, loss of sources of the self and social acceleration have meant that now, and accelerating ever more quickly, 'the biographical course of life as a whole loses *its direction*. It can no longer be understood as directed motion and narratively reconstructed in the sense of a history of progress and development. *Life doesn't head anywhere; in the end, it goes nowhere (very fast)*' (ibid.: 246, emphasis in the original). In accelerated late modern society,

> the inability (or unwillingness) to set temporally stable relevancies and to develop corresponding priorities of action in the sense of a 'task' that is built into the character of situational identity leads to a paradoxical inversion in which the experience of detemporalization, of temporal standstill, suddenly emerges out of the experience of 'temporalized' and so accelerated or 'racing' time.
>
> Ibid.

And suddenly we find that we have run out of time – life is simply 'game over'!

Conclusion

To conclude, we return to Weber's analysis of loss of *Beruf*, a vocation to a meaningful life task in service to an ideal. Today, Weber[12] says, *Beruf* has become secularized and rationalized into materialism, nihilism and the pursuit of wealth as an end in itself, but still in our thoroughly disenchanted world,

> the idea of duty in one's calling prowls around in our lives like the ghost of dead religious beliefs. Where the fulfilment of the calling [now devolved into simply 'earning a living'] cannot be related to the highest spiritual and cultural values, or when, on the other hand, it need not be felt as economic compulsion, the individual generally abandons any attempt to justify it at all.
>
> 1976/1905: 182

For some, the young perhaps, living life without a higher purpose, 'may begin to assume the character of a sport'; but as the game accelerates so that the rules are changing all the time, the goalposts suddenly shifting to a different, distant, always unsecure horizon, 'anxiety' becomes a characteristic individual pathology, for no matter how fit and flexible, how well-trained they may make themselves – assuming that they are, in fact, able to 'make themselves', given that the symbolic resources of the big Other are denied to them – playing the game successfully becomes increasingly difficult and for most, in the end, impossible. For more, somewhat older (and in what passes these days for a mid-stage career) people may have been willing to submit themselves to the structuring and ordering effects of the 'iron cage' of rationalized acquisitiveness, even if lack of higher cultural values and ideals have meant to become no more than 'specialists without spirit, hedonists without heart' (ibid.).

But desymbolization and social acceleration means that the cage has dissolved such that even the assurance of order and security of living within the cage is no longer a compensation for meaningless striving. The individual becomes freed from meaning-bearing and identity constituting social relations, becomes engaged in reflexive self-formation, though increasingly losing those institutional relations and symbolic orders that have until recently been available as sources of the self, and is faced with a new existential problem: this problem has been diagnosed – variously,

> first as *acedia*, then secularized as *melancholia*, as *ennui*, later as neurasthenia, and today as depression. In every case it is a matter of ... 'spiritual paralysis' in the face of the inability of the soul to direct its energy towards a fixed, constant, subjectively worthwhile goal and to express it in action.
>
> Rosa 2013: 249

Insecurities that had earlier been sources of anxiety now morph into 'depression':

> Depression is the handrail of the rudderless person. It is the reverse side of the expression of his energy.... this energy has insurmountable difficulties in unfolding productively when every possible relationship into which it can be invested will be transitory, passing, and hence not constitutive of identity.
>
> Ehrenberg, cited in ibid.

In an age of desymbolization and precarity, even those 'last men' who thought that they had 'invented happiness' become depressed![13] And for increasing numbers of people who experience the loss of even the conditions of possibility of having a vocation and of leading meaningful lives in accordance with their *Beruf*, we can interpret Alzheimer's disease and the dementia reputed to it in terms of how, in retrospect and in prospect, their lives have become incoherent, unmemorable and absurd. Just as anxiety is the modality of social pathology associated with racing time, and depression is the modality of social pathology associated with accelerated action without direction, dementia is the characteristic modality of social pathology of desymbolization, desynchronization and dissonance experienced by members of an aging population, who, disconnected and anxious, depressed and demented, drift away into the void.

Notes

1. The same is true of the 'biomarkers' of anxiety and depression. The ages of depression, anxiety and dementia are the 'age of the brain'. The *promise* of proof seems enough. 'It functions!'
2. The English edition has a different title, which is *Aging with Grace: The Nun Study and the Science of Old Age. How We Can All Live Longer, Healthier and More Vital Lives.* Apart from the title the books are verbatim. But the differences in the title are tremendously significant, and we shall use this as a way in to open up our understanding of Alzheimer's. In the first title our concern with Alzheimer's and the dementia reputed to it is articulated with the idea of life as being 'meaningful', but in the second case the idea of meaningfulness has been dropped out and replaced by the word 'vital'. The humanistic, philosophical, even sacred idea of the meaningfulness of life has been reduced to a profane biologistic matter of animal vitality. The reductive scientistic masterframe barges into the title as 'The Science of Old Age', elbowing aside the elderly nuns with their pedagogic vocation and what they may be able to 'teach' us.
3. See Szakolczai (2007) on the meanings and modalities of grace, charisma and gift.
4. For a comprehensive review and exposition of the literature see Baroncelli, (2014).
5. The etymology – *be rufen* – is 'to call', 'to be called', and the usage includes 'occupation', 'profession', 'trade', 'job', 'career'; encompassing also such uses as 'making a living' and having a 'talent', and thus a 'gift', a 'God-given gift'.
6. 'Malign', malignancy (from '*mal*' – meaning bad/evil and *gnus* – meaning birth/origin) and 'metastasis' (from 'meta' – to change and 'stasis' – to stand, means to change and spread rapidly to other places) are both terms that have a medical currency, especially in cancer, but also more generally in pathology, where they mean the tendency of disease to become progressively worse, affecting many vital systems and threatening the life of the entire organism.

7 The convent is one of Goffman's original exemplary cases.

8 The Durkheimian (sociological) concept of the *conscience collective* and the Lacanian (psychoanalytic) concept of the symbolic order are so congruent as to be practically synonymous: the *conscience collective* is a transcendent realm of 'social facts' to which the individual is subject – the big Other. In Durkheim's paradigm the collective representations (language, ideas, shared meanings) that constitute the *conscience collective* are 'the product of a vast cooperative effort that extends not only through space but over time; their creation has involved a multitude of different minds associating, mingling, combining their ideas and feelings – the accumulation of generations of experience and knowledge. A very special intellectuality, infinitely richer and more complex than that of the individual is concentrated in them' (Durkheim, 1995/1912;18). The *conscience collective* is 'a *sui generis* collective being formed by the plurality of individuals' minds' … 'something other than the totality of individuals that compose it' [simultaneously] 'something both beyond us and something in ourselves', 'a composition of ideas, beliefs and sentiments of all sorts which realize themselves through individuals' that 'transcends us and is immanent in us and we feel it as such' (Durkheim, 1974/1924: 51).

9 The periodization is somewhat arbitrary, as historical periodizations necessarily are, but we mean that complex whole of institutionalized social relationships that came to the fore in the aftermath of the democratic and industrial revolutions.

10 Add to this also the loss of structuring experiences of *rites de passage*, as traditional forms of life become dis-embedded, desynchronous and disintegrated under accelerating globalized modernization (Giddens 1991; Rosa 2013), and thus there are few meaning-making experiences of progressive status elevation for individuals through the life course, and few solidarity-building cohort experiences also. Life becomes increasingly and ever more rapidly individuated, randomized and characterized by 'permanent liminality' (Szakolczai 2000).

11 In which case, of course, that is not to say that the conditions of endemic dementia as a symptom of aged modernity cannot be ameliorated, for indeed they can, and this analysis, locating the sources of the problem in sociological conditions, is replete also with intimations of how the condition may be practically addressed. Here, for now, and simply as indicative, I will flag just one example that is in keeping with Rosa's diagnosis of the pathogenic effects of accelerated temporality as dysrhythmia and dissonance, namely: the design of Alzheimer's care centres as oases of deceleration, such as *De Hogeweyk* in Weesp, Holland, an Alzheimer's 'village' wherein the textures and rhythms of everyday life, down to the furnishings and décor and the music played on the radio – all of those things that constitute the tacitly assumed background and things that are 'ready to hand' – are carefully chosen so as to harmonize with the symbolic order and imaginative textures of residents' earlier familiar life-worlds in the 1950s and 1960s.

12 Weber is writing in 1905 or thereabouts, so it is prophetic of an aging civilization as well as diagnostic for a naively youthful modernity that has yet to experience even World War I.

13 In this context Weber says that 'after Nietzsche's devastating criticism of those "last men" who have "invented happiness", I may leave aside altogether the naïve optimism in which science – that is, the technique of mastering life which rests upon science – has been celebrated as the way to happiness. Who believes in this? – aside from a few big children in university chairs or editorial offices?' Perhaps also research directors of pharmaceutical companies chasing the 'cure' for Alzheimer's disease, not so much a happiness pill this time, but a 'meaningfulness' pill! Weber cites Dostoyevsky: 'Science is meaningless because it gives no answer to our question, the only question important for us: "What shall we do and how shall we live?"'

References

Antonovsky, A. (1987): *Unraveling the Mystery of Health: How People manage Stress and Stay Well.* San Francisco: Jossey-Bass.

Baroncelli Freitas, L. (2014): Depression and 'crises of meaninglessness' in the political-economic theology of the money-God. PhD dissertation, School of Sociology and Philosophy, University College Cork. Available online at: https://cora.ucc.ie/handle/10468/1971 (accessed 13 June 2016).

Blum, A. (2003): *The Imaginative Structure of the City.* Montreal: McGill-Queen's University Press.

Blum, A. (2012): The enigma of the brain and its place as cause, character and pretext in the imaginary of dementia. *History of the Human Sciences*, 25(4): 108–24.

Bourdieu, P. (1999): *Acts of Resistance: Against the Tyranny of the Market.* London: New Press.

Dejours, C. and Deranty, J.-P. (2010): The centrality of work. *Critical Horizons*, 11(2): 167–80.

Denning, T. and Thomas, A. (eds) (2013): *Oxford Textbook of Old Age Psychiatry.* Oxford: Oxford University Press.

Dufour, D.R. (2008): *The Art of Shrinking Heads: On the New Servitude of the Liberated in an Age of Total Capitalism.* Cambridge: Polity Press.

Dufour, D.R. (2011): *L'Individu Qui Vient … Après le Libéralisme.* Paris: Éditions Denoël.

Durkheim, E. (1974/1924): *Sociology and Philosophy.* New York: The Free Press.

Durkheim, E. (1995/1912): *The Elementary Forms of Religious Life.* New York: The Free Press.

Durkheim, E. (1997/1893): *The Division of Labour in Society.* New York: The Free Press.

Durkheim, E. (2002/1897): *Suicide.* London: Routledge.

Foucault, M. (1991): *Discipline and Punish: The Birth of the Prison.* London: Penguin.

Fratiglioni, L. and Hui-Xin, W. (2007): Brain reserve hypothesis in dementia. *Journal of Alzheimer's Disease*, 12(September): 11–22.

Giddens, A. (1991): *The Consequences of Modernity.* Cambridge: Polity Press.

Goffman, E. (1961): *Asylums: Essays on the Social Situation of Mental Patients and Other Inmates.* New York: Anchor Books.

Harvey, D. (2007): *A Brief History of Neoliberalism.* Oxford: Oxford University Press.

Ingram, J. (2014): *The End of Memory: A Natural History of Aging and Alzheimer's.* Toronto: HarperCollins.

Jameson, F. (1991): *Postmodernism, or The Cultural Logic of Late Capitalism.* Durham, NC: Duke University Press.

Kemper, S., Greiner, L.H., Marquis, J.G., Prenovost, K. and Mitzner, T.L. (2001): Language decline across the life span. *Psychology and Aging*, 16(2): 227–39.

Lock, M. (2013): *The Alzheimer Conundrum: Entanglements of Dementia and Aging.* Princeton, NJ: Princeton University Press.

Lyotard, J.F. (1984): *The Postmodern Condition: A Report on Knowledge.* Minneapolis: University of Minnesota Press.

Rosa, H. (2013): *Social Acceleration. A New Theory of Modernity.* New York: Columbia University Press.

Sennett, R. (1998): *The Corrosion of Character: The Personal Consequences of Work in the New Capitalism.* New York: Norton.

Snowdon, D. (2001): *Aging with Grace: What the Nun Study Teaches us about Leading Longer, Healthier, and More Meaningful Lives.* New York: Bantam Books (published simultaneously in the UK as *Aging with Grace: The Nun Study and the Science of Old Age. How We Can All Live Longer, Healthier and More Vital Lives.* London: Fourth Estate).

Szakolczai, A. (2000): *Reflexive Historical Sociology*. London: Routledge.

Szakolczai, A. (2007): *Sociology, Religion and Grace: A Quest for the Renaissance*. London: Routledge.

Taylor, C. (1989): *Sources of the Self: The Making of the Modern Identity*. Cambridge, MA: Harvard University Press.

Taylor, C. (1991): *The Ethics of Authenticity.* Cambridge, MA: Harvard University Press.

Taylor, C. (2007): *A Secular Age.* Cambridge, MA: Harvard University Press.

Turner, V. (1967): Betwixt and between: the liminal period in rites de passage. In: Turner, *The Forest of Symbols*. New York: Cornell University Press.

Weber, M. (1968/1919): Science as a vocation. In: Eisenstadt, S.N. (ed.), *Max Weber: On Charisma and Institution Building*. Chicago: University of Chicago Press.

Weber, M. (1976/1905): *The Protestant Ethic and the Spirit of Capitalism*. New York: Charles Scribner's Sons.

Weber, M. (1978/1919): 'Politics as a vocation'. In: Runciman, W.G. (ed.), *Max Weber: Selections in Translation*. Cambridge: Cambridge University Press.

6 A research prospective

Kieran Keohane, Anders Petersen and Bert van den Bergh

Social pathologies of contemporary civilization: symptomology and salutogenesis

Interregnum – from *inter* (between) and *regis* (king) – etymologically signifies the liminal period between the end of one sovereign power and the enthronement of another; a period during which – 'the old is dying and the new cannot be born; in this interregnum a great variety of morbid symptoms appear' (Gramsci 1971: 276). The interregnum of our present age is associated with an individual and collective experience of accelerating desymbolization: the loss of the names of the father, the decline of the power of master signifiers to constitute identity that integrate and morally regulate social life, the blurring of social norms and rules are generating a great variety of pathogenic effects, among them, as we have examined here, are anxiety, depression and dementia. Over the coming years we envisage a research programme in terms of a symptomology oriented to understanding and interpreting the many modalities of pathogenic accelerated desymbolization as they become ramified throughout the social and bodies politic, making themselves felt in individual and collective life at all levels. And beyond a critical-hermeneutic and phenomenological diagnostic symptomology, we are equally interested in exploring a therapeutics for recovery, for a holistic salutogenesis, a turning-around from the pathogenic currents pulsing and coursing through contemporary civilization, so that, in terms of Antonovsky's metaphor, we are not merely concerned with 'saving swimmers drowning downstream' or asking 'who or what is pushing them into the river in the first place', but even to reorienting the course of our collective socio-historical 'river of life', a river that has become very dangerous no matter how well one is able to swim.

Historical *ricorso* and pathologies of civilization

The circulation of social pathogenic 'currents' and salutogenic 'rivers of life' brings us immediately into conversation with Giambattista Vico's philosophy of history as *ricorso*, presented in *Scienza Nuova* as an interpretation of the rise and fall of ancient civilizations as recorded in mythology and poetics. There are 'two great maladies' during periods that precede recurring dark ages, Vico says: 'the perfect tyranny of anarchy and the unbridled liberty of free peoples' (1999/1744: 487). In our contemporary period, a mythic age of globalized modernity accelerating to hypermodernity; an age of desymbolization and post-modernism, the mythic age of the neoliberal revolution – these maladies appear as the anarchy of the deregulated Market and the 'liberation' of the subject from the Name of the Father. In response to these two maladies of civilization, three patterns of social action recur historically, Vico says. The first is the restoration of internal monarchy by a charismatic demagogue who restores order by powerful violence – a form of politics we see recurring throughout Europe and America today. A second recurring pattern is that societies weakened by such maladies become subject to conquest by external powers, which can be seen today in the eclipsing of the sovereignty of nation states and their public goods of social security, education and health care, by market forces – ownership and rule by a global dynasty of private transnational corporate despotic plutocrats. And the third recurring historical pattern of social action is that we become bestial again – solitary, competitive, un-cooperative, 'living like beasts, crowded together but divided amongst ourselves' (ibid.). Tendencies towards all three characterize the contemporary *zeitgeist*.

Speaking of another moment of historical *ricorso*, a period with striking resemblances to our own, Hannah Arendt (2006/1963) says that the banality of evil was not Fascism or Communism but the moral failure of European civilization as a whole, its fall to immanence and nihilism and the genesis of a new kind of non-thinking subject. Today, ultraliberalism that celebrates and promotes Hobbesian free market anarchy means that we become a mob of private individuals, crowded together but divided among ourselves; born-again Cyclopes, glowering from the mouths of our caves. Lost to the collective life of society, we fall as individuals into a void of chaos, which, according to Vico, is the original monster, Orcus, that devours men whole. Hermes can call souls back from the dead, Vico says. Hermes the communicator 'carries the law … calls souls back from Orcus, meaning he calls back to society those who were again dispersed in the lawless state of barbarism that devours men whole' (Vico 1999/1744: 168). Hermes can 'call us back' from chaos, Vico says, so it's not that we need a new law/ruling principle/Name of the Father – that we have to imagine entirely new names of the father; but rather that we need to remember/recollect/recall, 'call back', 'turn around' – actually to reimagine, for 'imagination is simply the resurfacing of recollections and ingenuity is simply the elaboration of things remembered' (ibid.: 315). Similarly, Walter Benjamin, for instance, talks about memory and renewal in terms of digging into the past, 'returning again and again to the same matter; to scatter it as one scatters earth, to turn it over as one turns over soil, finding in the rich loam the real treasures hidden within the earth' (Benjamin 1977: 314). Because everything becomes buried with the passage of time 'in every era the attempt must be made anew to wrest tradition away from the conformism that is about to overpower it' (Benjamin 1992: 247).

Expressing these ideas of memory, imagination and redeeming buried treasures in the language of contemporary social and political thought, Charles Taylor (2007: 748) says:

> All valid ideals are already anchored in a deep tradition, in ways of life which have already been lived. They cannot enter history like a newly invented plan that sweeps reality aside or shapes it from above. The validly new is a recreation of a tradition.

Chantal Mouffe emphasizes the radical emancipatory potential in this reinvented, reimagined tradition:

> Tradition allows us to think of our own insertion into historicity, the fact that we are constructed as subjects through a series of already existing discourses, that it is through this tradition that forms us that the world is given to us and all political action made possible.
>
> Mouffe 1988: 39

As 'tradition' is the set of discourses and practices that form us as subjects, we should think of politics as:

> the pursuit of intimations within those discourses … which in a Wittgensteinian perspective can be understood as the creation of new usages for the key terms of a given tradition, and of their use in new language games that make new forms of life possible.
>
> Ibid.: 41

And, most recently, concerning the need for recollection, Dany-Robert Dufour has emphasized the distinction – referring to Freud and Marcuse – between necessary and unnecessary repression: the latter concerns the subjection of the other and needs to be contested, the former relates to the disciplining of the passions and is connected to an extensive tradition that we need to guard and recall. For a long time, Dufour writes in *L'Individu Qui Vient … Après le Libéralisme*, the leading thought was that, in order to beat capitalism, one has to become revolutionary. 'This is a capital mistake: *the only truly revolutionary regime is capitalism*' (Dufour 2011: 303, emphasis in the original). The only way to resist capitalism is to refuse the permanent revolution of social relations it brings about. How? By becoming reactionary or conservative? No, by developing a narrative that Dufour terms *neo-resistant* and *conservatoire*, neo-resistant and conserving. It is crucial for us to make the distinction between acting conservingly and being conservative:

> One should not revolutionize *everything*, as the Market presently wants us to believe, one should *only* revolutionize the places where secondary or additional repressions exist (those which proletarize men and control

> women), so places that correspond to an inappropriate confiscation of enjoyment [*jouissance*, ed.]. But one should also *conserve* the necessary primary repression which obliges everybody to endure a withdrawal of enjoyment from his/her possible pleonexic tendencies and potential egoistic inclinations. And if this already has been destroyed by the Market and one is too late to conserve, one should undertake a *restauration*.
>
> Ibid.: 306, emphasis in the original

Metanoia and metaphor

If the powerful current of the present historical *ricorso* is not to suck us into Orcus's abysmal depths, what is needed is nothing short of individual and collective metanoia, and the metaphors that may bring that about.

Metanoiein (Greek) means 'to change one's mind' (from *meta-* after, beyond, and *noein* to think, from *nous* mind). The corona of shades of meanings in the semantic field of words that bear family resemblances to metanoia include 'transmutation', 'transfiguration', 'metamorphosis' and 'metempsychosis' (in the sense of being taken over, becoming possessed and animated by powerful spirits). Metanoia means 'a change in the trend and action of the whole inner nature, intellectual, affectional and moral'; a 'transmutation of consciousness'; 'transfiguration – a complete change of form into a higher and more beautiful state' (Merriam-Webster; *Oxford English Dictionary*). Metanoia is associated with regeneration and rebirth, with renaissance. Metanoia means 'conversion' – that is, being 'turned' – 'turned around' in a completely different direction, 'turned towards' sources of illumination, radiant ideals that lead us in a higher moral and spiritual direction. This accords with Plato's famous definition in *Republic* of education as the turning of the soul (518 c–d). Where one had been going astray, metanoia means finding the proper direction, finding one's true vocation – *Beruf*, 'calling', with all of the moral-practical and political connotations, intimations and resonances of *Beruf* as 'vocation'/calling, with the notion of illumination by the light of radiant ideals. So, what metanoia has come to mean today has a long genealogy, from classical philology, through theology, to psychology and to pedagogy; a genealogy showing a progressive deepening of meaning, from an original usage signifying a relatively superficial change of mind, as in 'to change one's opinion' about a particular matter or point of view, to metanoia used 'to express that mighty change in mind, heart, and life wrought by the Spirit of God' (Trench 2006: 260). And there is a cluster of significations associated with Metanoia as personified in Greek and Roman mythology, as a spirit of repentance and regret. Metanoia is twinned with the spirit of Kairos – the spirit of opportunity. The spirit of Metanoia follows behind Kairos, where she laments missed opportunity – in other words, metanoia is when a crisis, for example, presents us also with an opportunity, but we fail to see it and to seize it at the crucial moment, and we have a change of heart and mind only when it is already too late, when the opportunity to do the right thing has already passed (Myers 2011).

Metanoia in psychology, pedagogy and politics

William James (1890) uses metanoia to refer to a fundamental and stable change in an individual's life-orientation. In Jung's (1960) usage metanoia refers to the mind's attempt to heal itself of unbearable conflict by melting down (as in a mental breakdown) and then re-emerging, reborn in a more adaptive form. For Jung, psychotic breaks in particular should be understood in terms of existential crises and attempted self-healing, a theme taken up by contemporary radical psychiatry (R.D. Laing) and in (Freudian, and Lacanian) psychoanalysis also, wherein the modalities of mental breakdown may manifest as anxiety and depression – anxiety as the person's former reality disintegrates; depression as grieving for the lost loved object, lost by virtue of metanoia.

For Charles Taylor (1991: 84) metanoia means 'to change one's mind and attitude', a fundamental change in perception, understanding and mind. In Taylor's formulation the centre of Jesus's ministry was a call to metanoia, a transformative change of heart; especially, a spiritual conversion. Metanoia, thus, is the central thing that needs to happen to bring about change, whether in the realm of religion/spirituality, or in pedagogy, or in politics – that the deeper meaning of 'conversion', 'learning' and of 'leading' is metanoia. Metanoia as 'a change of perception with its behavioral fruit' (ibid.) resonates strongly with Nietzsche's '*Umwertung*', with Heidegger's '*Kehre*', with Wittgenstein's 'aspect viewing' and with Walter Benjamin's notion of 'dialectical image' as '*Denkbilder*', and it is with these resonances that we now attune ourselves, in order to prepare ourselves for a fundamental retunement.

Metaphor as method: aesthetic ideas, *Denkbilder* and language games

Ontology and epistemology are grounded in language and communication; beyond merely using signifiers and signified, we make sense and convey meaning, we transcend the givenness of the world, we reach beyond, we create – and we imaginatively re-create – our world, by use of metaphors.

> The drive toward the formation of metaphors is the fundamental human drive, which one cannot for a single instant dispense with in thought, for one would thereby dispense with man himself …
>
> What then is truth? A movable host of metaphors, metonymies, and anthropomorphisms: in short, a sum of human relations which have been poetically and rhetorically intensified, transferred, and embellished, and which, after long usage, seem to a people to be fixed, canonical, and binding. Truths are illusions that we have forgotten are illusions.
>
> Nietzsche 1882/1873: 46–7

Metaphors, Kant says, can enable us to transcend the limits of both pure reason and practical reason and help 'to bring reason into harmony with itself' (Kant 2002/1875: 49).

> By an aesthetical Idea [Kant speaks about metaphors, allegories and similes used in poetic, mythic and religious language, in visual arts, music, film, dance, dramatic performance, literature and poetry] I understand that representation of the imagination which occasions much thought, without, however, any definite thought, *i.e.* any *concept*, being capable of being adequate to it; it consequently cannot be completely compassed and made intelligible by language.... Such representations of the Imagination we may call *Ideas*, partly because they at least strive after something that lies beyond the bounds of experience.
>
> Ibid., emphasis in the original

Metaphors have transformative power because they help us to strain out beyond the confines of experience in the world towards what is beyond the world – they give us glimpses of an ideal realm of Beauty, Truth and the Good.

And in the Lacanian paradigm: meaning is an effect of the signifying chain; contingent upon discourse; upon 'hegemonic articulatory practices' (Laclau and Mouffe, 1985). Master signifiers that (purport to) fix the flow of signification lend things the semblance of truth, but are themselves underpinned by the real, that is to say by the lack of ultimate ground. As Geertz (citing Weber) says: 'we are suspended in webs of signification that only we ourselves have spun' (1973: 5). The web of language covering the void is pinned together by powerful metaphors within which meaning is condensed and concentrated: such metaphors are the authoritative name(s) of the father. Biopsychiatry, the nosology of the *DSM*, the simple facts of neurochemistry are among those authorities that claim to pin down anxiety, depression and Alzheimer's disease and other malaises of contemporary civilization. But,

> the pinning down I speak of, or the *point de capiton* is mythical, for no one has been able to pin a signification on a signifier; but on the other hand what can be done is to pin one signifier to another signifier and see what happens. In this case something new is invariably produced ... in other words the surging forth of a new signification.
>
> Lacan 1991: 274

Producing new significations, new meanings and new understandings is the work performed by metaphors. 'The creative spark of the metaphor ... flashes between two signifiers one of which has taken the place of the other in the signifying chain' (Lacan 1977: 156–7).

Walter Benjamin would say of these formulations of our ontology and epistemology from Nietzsche, from Kant and from Lacan that late modernity/post-modernity/hypermodernity, far from being an escape from mythic domination through Enlightenment is, in fact, a further extension and elaboration of mythic consciousness (Gilloch 1997), a dream of reason, a fantasy of progress; that, like the Greeks and other ancient and non-Modern cultures, we continue to be a mythically inspired people, and we will not break free of myth by virtue of Enlightenment and the power of reason alone, for this 'dream of reason'[1] itself is part of the conceit! Rather, the way through myth, the way to 'show the fly the way to escape from the bottle' in Wittgenstein's idiom, is 'to change the aspect under which the thing is viewed'; in Benjamin's terms 'to use myth against myth', to introduce new metaphors, to give new meanings to the key terms of the prevailing language games so that the character and the trajectory of the narrative is turned around, effecting a metanoia that is at once subjective – psychological and collective – sociological-historical and moral-political. Hermes is the spirit of politics, of communication, the God of metaphor, the God of carrying over (Hyde, 1998). As psychopomp, he carries souls from one realm to the next; in other words, he carries the 'spirit', the 'sense', the 'meaning' from one thing to another (Graves 1960; Kerenyi 1980).

In this sense, as Vico says, it is by the political use of metaphor that we can be turned around and called back from chaos and barbarism, for metaphor is where the arts of poetics and rhetoric intersect to create persuasive new insights (Ricoeur 1993). Such use of metaphor to bring about a transformative metanoia is what Benjamin has in mind when he says somewhere that his *Denkbilder* are as tools in the hands of a knowledgeable and skilful engineer, by means of which he need make only a small adjustment that will change the whole direction and operation of the huge machine. And to update Benjamin's analogue metaphor so as to attune with today's digital technologies, we may speak of a meme – an idea, behaviour or style that spreads from person to person within a culture. A meme acts as a hermetic device for carrying ideas, symbols, or practices that can be transmitted from one mind to another through writing, speech, gestures, rituals, or other imitable phenomena with a mimicked theme. As in a previous – and still prescient – register full of similar resonances, Donna Haraway (1989) uses the notion of a 'viral vector': in the cyborg world of digital-biological interfaces effected by neurogenetic and nano-engineering, aesthetic images – metaphors as internet memes – may act as viral vectors, hermetic keys that we may send back through the matrix in such a way as to re-code it. Against the pathogenic 'inscription of a digital rhythm on the social body' Berardi identifies a dialectical interior counter-rhythm in terms of a 'rhizomatic poetics of insurrection', 'of slowness, withdrawal … the autonomization of the collective body and soul from the exploitation of speed and competition' (2012: 29, 68).

'To imagine a language is to imagine a form of life,' Wittgenstein says; in other words, the language we use when we talk about something – which frames, perceives and understands, grasps and expresses – constitutes a 'language game', a meaningful and meaning-giving 'whole, consisting of language and the actions into which it is woven'. The prevailing language game, within which there may be numerous pathways, flows and confluences – political-economic and cultural, and with numerous national and regional variations bearing family resemblances to one another – constitutes the reality of world; for nothing exists – there can be no meaningful world – outside of language (Wittgenstein 1994/1958: 7. – And Beckett too, of course, who says that outside of language there is nothingness: silence, madness and death). Thus, to make a Wittgensteinian corollary, if we are to imagine a different world, a better form of life – then we must imagine a different language: we need to develop and learn to play new language game(s).

We are trapped within the prevailing language game. In our being subject to this language game (we might also say discursive, or cognitive frame), we are 'like a fly trapped in a bottle'; and the task is twofold: first to shake and disrupt the prevailing language games within which we are trapped – the hegemony of the biopsychiatric diagnostic individual reductive master frame foremost among them, connected to the neoliberal newspeak of 'resilience' and 'empowerment' – and also 'to show the fly the way out of the bottle', by 'changing the aspect under which things are viewed' (ibid.: 309, 195–6). How can we get a perspective on our situation by virtue of which we may be able to imagine alternatives?

Aspect viewing, remembering and reimagining

Sociological imagination, C. Wright Mills (1959) says, is a method of looking at the world as through a lens or a prism with many facets. As well as working within the sociological paradigm, with its often contrasting perspectives, one should actively seek anthropological perspectives, historical perspectives, philosophical (i.e. ideal) perspectives; perspectives from poetry, literature and the arts; perspectives from mythology and from theology; insights from self-reflective autobiographical, biographical and psychoanalytic perspectives; perspectives from etymology, philology comparative linguistics and semiotics; and others too. 'Try to think in terms of a variety of viewpoints and in this way to let your mind become a moving prism catching light from as many angles as possible' (ibid.: 214). By this means of aspect viewing we can think ourselves away from the restrictions of our prevailing language games/semantic fields/discursive regimes of truth, and look on problems of our own reality from different points of view.

Mills' prism for Wittgensteinian aspect viewing for problem-solving is an imaginative sociological method for addressing the social pathologies of contemporary civilization. Method, from *hodos* (a path, a road), means a 'way', a way of going about something; a *Weg* Heidegger would say, using the metaphor of a 'pathway' in the forest, a forest pathway that lies 'near at hand', that, if we follow it, will lead us to a 'clearing' wherein we may pause, reflect, take our bearings and 'see the wood for the trees', as it were. Anthropologically and historically, pathways, paths that eventually become roads, run alongside rivers; rivers have been civilizations' highways; so that by virtue of the world's rivers we have passage and portage, 'crossing', 'ferrying', 'carrying over'. Metaphor, from *meta* (beyond, over, across) and *pherein* (to carry, to bear, to transport) means 'carrying over', 'carrying across', 'conveying' 'transferring', and Hermes – spirit of the messenger, spirit of transit, spirit of the crossroads – is the spirit of finding a way. Meaning is carried over by metaphor, enabling thinking and doing, being and living to go on as a collective sociological and moral form of life. A metaphor is Hermes as a porter carrying a baggage of meanings; conveying a portmanteau of values, goods exchanged in the commerce of communication as the stock in trade that enables meaning-making to continue its journey, as a caravan, a train of thought, a stream of consciousness, an aesthetic – therapeutic narrative … a walking-talking cure.

In what follows we will draw out some extended metaphors/*Denkbilder* that have something to show us about a diagnostics and therapeutics of the social pathologies of contemporary civilization.

Horizon, transgression and liminality

Orcus (Roman), Horkos (Greek), whom we have met already, is a primordial demon who punishes oath-breakers. Orcus devours men whole, which means that, without oaths – Laws – that govern and limit human action in the Name of the Father, we descend into chaos and barbarism (Vico 1999/1744: 688). Orcus establishes limits; his name is derived from *horos*, meaning 'boundaries of regions and territories'. In mythology and etymology, Orcus/Horkos becomes Horion/Orion (from which we have 'horizon', limit): Orion is a mortal hero; he crosses boundaries and transcends limits. Orion is the first hunter; he shows us how to kill – the first great transgression! But because he knows no limits he is in danger of killing all the animals on Earth. Hedonistic, free, driven only by his passions, Orion gets drunk and has sex with his own mother. Orion befriends the gods, but he has no traffic with his fellow human beings; he is not anthropologically grounded in any social community. He has sex with the goddess Artemis and then with Apollo, her brother. The three had previously been friends, but now the boundary of friendship has been crossed; a friends and siblings' relationship becomes a jealously charged *ménage à trois*. Knowing no bounds, no regulations, Orion violates taboos, transgresses limits – both human and divine. He scrambles all boundaries, causing confusion and trouble because of his ungoverned passions, his hubris and pleonexia (Kerenyi 1980: 204–5). *Pleonexia* is excessive and insatiable greed, vaulting ambition and envy, lust for money, power and honour, within a broader historical political-economic context of gross social inequality and unfairness. For three millennia there had been a general consensus across theology, philosophy, ethics, politics and even medicine that pleonexia was a social pathology. Insatiability was always a sign of morbidity, both in the case the individual with raging appetites and in social and bodies politic. Socrates, Plato and Aristotle all identify pleonexia as the root cause of the collapse of Athenian civilization. Thucydides agrees, and Livy also in the case of the decline and fall of Rome. But modern liberalism – and neoliberalism especially – makes a virtue of pleonexia – 'greed is good'! Pleonexia is a latent pathology, as it is anthropologically deep-seated in human nature, in our animal appetites and instincts, repressed and contained in the unconscious by the social super-ego; but it can become manifest under certain conditions. Ordinarily limited, governed, mediated and sublimated, pleonexia flourishes as symptomatic social pathologies during liminal historical periods of accelerated social and political transformation during which there are dissolutions and mutations of the symbolic order.

People tend to become extravagantly acquisitive, over-reaching in their ambitions, suspicious and aggressively envious of others when the normal constraints and limits that govern and contain individual appetites and desires are loosened and become uncertain. Pleonexia cannot be contained when there is no certainty, no consensus on the principles according to which distribution should take place. In such circumstances 'the powerful do what they can, and the weak suffer what they must', as Thucydides says. When the individual is not beholden to previously prevailing norms and conventions and there is lack of answerability to collective principles, when the social super-ego is lacking, pleonexia is a social pathology of unrestrained egoism and narcissism that can tend towards psychosis (Balot 2001a, 2001b; Thomassen 2013).[2]

As an embodiment of pleonexia and hubris, Orion is an archetype/prototype, historical recurrence of the Sadean isolist neoliberal subject. By erasing limits, deregulating all boundaries and by being killed by Apollo and Artemis together for doing so, Orion stands also for the need to establish new limits in contexts where limits have been transgressed and regulations erased. The gods hung out Orion's body in the sky as a constellation, so that by gazing to the heavens we may remember the moral lesson that the story of Orion teaches us.[3]

In the mythology of Orion we have a genealogy of the big Other in Classical civilization, and in this source we can also see how high the stakes are when the symbolic order is shaken and scrambled, which is nothing less than a crisis of civilization of world-historical consequence. In the processes of accelerating deregulation and desymbolization wrought by the global neoliberal revolution, we can see a repetition of these mythic themes, especially at the level of political anthropology, namely in the mutation of the post-modern subject. We are approaching the event horizon of a new dark age – perhaps it is already upon us?

'The oldest of the old follows behind us in our thinking, and yet it comes to meet us,' Heidegger (1971: 10). Under the auspices of the neoliberal revolution individualism has reached a new stage, where a post-social subject increasingly sees him/herself as a self-creator. The neoliberal subject is the return of Orion again, one who is subject to no authority, one who acknowledges no limits. How will the new Orion (that is to say, how will we) find ways of limiting ourselves lest the gods kill us and scatter our ashes to the universe as stardust? For all of his excess, Orion is a mortal human being. He is talented and beautiful, strong and heroic, a splendid, self-realizing, autonomous individual. Artemis and Apollo both love him, before his insatiability and his vanity become the death of him. As much as he is a transgressive pleonexic monster, Orion is a tragic and a sympathetic figure. The essence of his problem is that he has not agreed to give anything up so he can be part of society, which is, precisely, the psychoanalytic formulation of psychosis (Salecl 2011: 68). Because Orion cannot sacrifice his desire, subject himself to any name(s) of the father, confine himself within the horizons of normal social limits, he suffers: he is megalomaniacal, out of control, a wild man; even his own mother cannot trust him not to rape her. Suffering psychosis, Orion is alone, vulnerable and anxious; he needs his mother's love, he needs the friendship of the gods and he experiences if not remorse, then at least confusion and bewilderment when he has set Artemis and Apollo against one another and they contrive to kill him. Orion shows us the horizon of danger where grounds and limits are lacking; where pleonexic energies are unleashed; where grounds and limits are needed.

Cardiology of contemporary civilization: heart of darkness revisited

The combined effects of desymbolization – the erosion of the authority of master signifiers and meaning-giving Enlightenment and modern metanarratives that authorize (or that sanction) social action 'in the name(s) of the father(s)'- and social acceleration to hypermodernity means that we have lost contact with structure (sociological and anthropological structures and institutions, and extending even to ontological and epistemological structure). On the one hand, we have been losing anthropological foundations in the sense of generalized consciousness of common origins and mutual deep human needs and, on the other hand and at the same time, we are suffering from a loss of limits, in the sense of social/moral horizons defined by shared transcendent ideals. The collective simultaneous loss of contact with structure in terms of both anthropological grounds and of philosophical-sociological/moral-political transcendent limits generates dysrhythmia and dissonance, for, seeking to find ground and limit by transgression and excess, we oscillate wildly to extremes. Resonance (and rhythm) is an oscillation between ground and limit; dissonance (and dysrhythmia) is when there is no limit, or no ground, so there can be no reverberation, no resonance. We need to find rhythm and resonance and thus recover the possibility of social harmony grounded in empathic understanding of deep human needs and shared commitment to transcendent ideals.

Recent terror attacks in Paris/London/Brussels – 'the heart of Europe' – are occasions to reflect upon dissonance and dysrhythmia as a diagnostics of the social pathologies of contemporary civilization and to develop a metaphor of cardiology in the social and bodies politic. To work with cardiology is to take up one of the most ancient medical arts,[4] which is taking the pulse, listening to the heartbeat, attuning to the patient – an attuning that reunites divisions and dichotomies of modernity, namely the dualism of 'head' (reason/mind) and 'heart' (passion/body) from the Cartesian epistemology of *cogito ergo sum* and the reversal/inversion in contemporary medicine whereby *psyche* is eclipsed by *soma*. We must think and speak in terms of holistic health and collective psychosomatics – biology and psychiatry reconciled, not by reducing the focus to individuated cytology and neurology of biochemical selves but rather at the level of the symbolic order and the imaginative structures within which the person is a member of the living collective organism as a moral totality.

To take up the metaphor of cardiology is to pay attention to circulation, to flows and currents, of which three stand out especially: revenue flows from citizens as debtors, to creditors – banks and bondholders, and from there to off-shore tax havens – cold digitized cash flows of which the digital-commercial river of Amazon, with its diversions from all tributary national revenue streams, is one example. A second current is the cooling Gulf Stream, symptomatic of anthropogenic global climate change, a deathly planetary hyperthermia caused by feverish production and consumption. The third circulation is a flow of shivering human bodies, migrants and refugees, from Africa, the Middle East and Asia. Durkheim associated the suicidogenic currents that flowed and pulsed and swirled through modern European societies with older and deeper sea-changes of the moral foundations and symbolic orders of European civilization that were the Enlightenment, and before that the Reformation and the Renaissance, as in our time we have late (or post-) modernity and the neoliberal revolution as pathological currents that pulse and swirl down the rivers of life and across the seas of the world; today's global currents of Transatlantic and Trans-Pacific ('free') Trade and Investment 'partnerships'; of refugees' bodies washing up on Mediterranean beaches; of the weakening Gulf Stream heralding apocalypse for an overheated planet in the form of a second flood: we live in a new antediluvian moment.

The journey up the river slicked with rubber and blood into modernity's 'heart of darkness' is narrated from a boat on the Thames, waiting for the tide to turn, reverberating with a voyage 2,000 years previously and the flood and ebb of Roman civilization. Kurtz, the protagonist of *Heart of Darkness*, is an early incarnation of neoliberalism's *homo economicus* as Sadean libertine isolist.[5] 'All Europe contributed to the making of Kurtz,' Conrad (2009/1899: 54) says. He is western civilization in short (*kurz* is German for 'short'). Kurtz is purported to be a 'great man', a 'universal genius' with 'immense plans'. He eloquently expounds on all the ideals of Enlightenment and modernity – development, growth, progress – but 'he had kicked himself loose of the Earth' (ibid.: 72). 'His intelligence was perfectly clear – concentrated, it is true, upon himself with horrible intensity... images of wealth and fame revolving obsequiously round his inextinguishable gift of noble and lofty expression. My intended, my station, my career, my ideas' (ibid.: 74). Kurtz seems to be a subject of reason but he is 'a hollow sham' his 'method is unsound'; 'Mr Kurtz lacked restraint in the gratification of his various lusts,... there was something wanting in him' (ibid.: 63). The project of modern civilization that he represents – *laissez faire* economic liberal individualism – falls short: Kurtz is a creature of the modern jungle, an isolist who has gone beyond; transgression as a way of life has brought him back – or forwards again – to the barbarism of a state of nature. Kurtz is diseased, his malaria marks him as the walking dead;[6] the post-social living dead, incapable of caring for others, even others of its own kind, the pleonexic, amoral, acritical, ahistorical Sadean isolist libertine.

Kurtz personifies the impossibility or un-liveability of the Sadean position – detached; detuned; deranged. In De Sade's narrative 'all creatures struggle only for their own survival and supremacy' (in Hallam 2012: 45). In this De Sade is perfectly in tune with contemporary neoliberalism: 'survival of the fittest'; a monstrous ideal of abstract animal power (Ransom 1939: 318). Here we have a slavery that goes way beyond that of the exploitation of the powerless by the powerful. Here we have the self-destruction of the self-imprisoning pleonexic. 'This is the dead land/this is cactus land', T.S. Eliot wrote in 'The Hollow Men' (1991: 80). This is the heart of darkness in contemporary civilization.

Dissonance: sounding contemporary civilization's hollow icons

There is a frightful dissonance between Kurtz's words – his 'inexhaustible gift for lofty expression', and his deeds – his complete amorality; 'he has kicked himself free of the Earth', a freedom that has made him 'unsound'.

> Freedom of trade is complete in the Congo, and is restricted neither by monopoly nor privilege. Every one is free to sell or buy every sort of produce in which it is lawful to trade. The law protects this freedom by forbidding any interference with the freedom of business transactions; it punishes any one who has employed violence or threats with a view to compel the natives, whether on the roads in the interior, or in the markets, to part with their goods to particular persons or at particular prices; it punishes those who, by violence, abuse, or threats, shall, have interfered with the freedom of trade, with a view either to stop trade caravans on the public roads or to obstruct the freedom of traffic whether by land or water.
>
> *Bulletin Official de l'Etat Independent du Congo*, cited in Casement 1904: 17

Whereas this is the rhetoric of the ideal in the Congo Free State, Roger Casement's soundings reveal an entirely dissonant reality:

> August 6th: Took copious notes from natives … they are cruelly flogged for being late with their baskets.
>
> August 13th … five people from Bokoro side with hands cut off had come as far as Myanga to show me.
>
> August 29th: Bogandanga … saw rubber 'market', nothing but guns … Poplin.[7]
>
> Two hundred and forty two men with rubber, all guarded like convicts. To call this 'trade' is the height of lying.

> August 30th: Sixteen men women and children tied up from a village Myobe … Infamous. Infamous. Shameful system!
>
> Casement, cited in Hochschild 1998: 202

In the Amazon Casement finds the same dissonance between the rhetoric representing the hollow idol of 'free trade' and the reality of 'slavery without law or limit'.

> It must always be borne in mind that the Indian is no party to the contract. He is compelled by brutal and wholly uncontrolled force – by being hunted and caught – by floggings, by chaining up, by long periods of imprisonment and starvation, to agree to 'work' for the Company, and then when released from this taming process and his 5/[shillings] worth of absolute trash given to him he is hunted and hounded and guarded and flogged and his food robbed and his womenfolk ravished until he brings in from 200 to perhaps 300 times the value of the goods he has been forced to accept (Casement 1997/1910: 216).
>
> The whole thing from top to bottom is slavery without law – the most lawless state of things imaginable in this stage of human progress, for these Agents are not savages, but are the highly paid servants of a great English Company – citizens of a civilized state and amenable, so we are told, to an 'Efficient administration of justice' (Sunday, 30th October 1910).
>
> Casement ibid: 174

We can hear resonances of this today in the dissonance between the rhetoric and the reality of the new generation of 'free trade' deals, namely TTIP (Transatlantic Trade and Investment Partnership), TPP (Trans-Pacific Partnership) and CETA (Comprehensive Economic and Trade Agreement).

> What they want is stripping away regulations. Harmonizing down. They're not saying, okay let's harmonize standards on intellectual property to make access to generic medicines more accessible for everybody, that will lower the price, and that will improve health care. That's not what they're talking about. They're talking about … a way of making drug prices high, or reducing access to generic medicine, extending for biologics to 12 years. Even President Obama opposes that. But his trade minister, the USTR [US Trade Representative] is taking a position that is extreme even for the United States, and insisting on that for TPP and TTIP. So that's harmonizing to a standard that is in the advantage of big pharma against American people, European people, generics, access to health. So we wouldn't have that if we had and open debate in Congress and in the European Parliament. They would not accept this. It's being done this way because the big pharma knows it can't get it through our parliament, through our Congress. And it's using an end run, in secret, to get around democratic processes.
>
> Stiglitz 2015

The flag of the Congo Free State, a gold star on blue background, suggested by H.M. Stanley to Leopold II to represent 'the bright star of Western Civilization bringing light to darkest Africa', celebrates 'free trade' as Casement found it to be above. This theme is echoed in today's flag of Europe – 12 gold stars on blue background, a design inspired by the diadem of the Madonna of the Apocalypse in Strasburg Cathedral, or, sourced from a different mythology, the 12 stars representing balance and perfection, the cosmos of the 12 gods of Olympus.[8]

Walking with, talking through: towards a walking-talking cure

When Roger Casement goes into the heart of the Congo, by listening to the natives, recording, reporting, he is 'sounding' the icons of western civilization, 'modernity', 'mankind', 'progress' and, especially, 'free trade'. Casement is looking for resonance in the ideals of contemporary civilization, but he finds them hollow, empty rhetoric. Casement's reports are a practical and moral-political case of what Nietzsche calls 'philosophizing with a hammer', the crushing of *Götze*, false gods, idols. The rhetoric of 'European civilization', 'progress' and 'free trade' ring hollow to his soundings, and the dissonance Casement experiences between the ideals and the realities become the basis of his own personal metanoia, his transformation of consciousness and the turning of his character onto a new path … from his being British Consul, His Majesty's Loyal Servant, to his becoming an Irish republican revolutionary who would eventually be hanged for High Treason. During his Congo journey, walking and talking and bearing witness with the Congolese, Casement says that he came to view the world from a different aspect:

> I realized then that I was looking at this tragedy with the eyes of another race, of a people once hunted themselves … And I said to myself, there, far up the Lulonga river, that I would do my part as an Irishman wherever it might lead me to personally.
>
> Casement, in Hochschild 2012: 268

Casement walks alongside the Congolese and the Putumayo Indians; he listens to them; he talks with them; he bears witness.[9] Casement travels by boat and by train too, but mostly he walks, back along the rivers, towards the sources of the trouble he sees downstream, the rivers of ivory and rubber, slaves and blood. While walking, by walking alongside the porters, he bears witness; he observes; he listens; he talks; he records what he sees and hears; he reports (re-ports – carries back, carries over, to the Foreign Office, to the general public, to contemporary people). Casement has qualities of Hermes – he is eloquent, a charming and gifted communicator. A gay cosmopolitan, a child of Hermes and Aphrodite, Casement is an erotic and promiscuous spirit. Everyone found Casement to be an impressive talker. 'His greatest charm was his voice, which was very musical' (Hochschild 2012: 197).

Crisis and *kairos*: rivers of migrants, rivers of life …

Today, the 'crisis' of the so-called 'river' of refugees and migrants, that many say 'threatens' to 'flood' Europe, if viewed from a different aspect, if articulated in a different language game, can be seen and expressed in terms of *kairos*, as a golden opportunity for contemporary civilization to recall the ideals that give it its *raison d'être* and its *telos*, radiant ideals that have been lost sight of, that have become faded and obscured; ideals that had deep resonance, but that are being systematically undermined and hollowed out by processes of social acceleration and desymbolization. By a moral-political intervention (that is, by reframing and reimagining the refugee 'crisis' by virtue of the interpretive arts of Hermes) we may be able to seize an opportunity to effect a metanoia; a turning-around of the situation so that grounds that have been undermined and ideals that have become hollowed out and lost sight of to us can become unconcealed, made resonant, and brought to light through a *poiesis* of our being-with the Other, rediscovering again our mutual vulnerability and our common deep need for care.

Floodplains and watersheds are the birthplaces of civilization because floodplains are fertile – the three great monotheistic religions, Jewish, Christian and Islamic, the confluences and divergences of whose streams have flowed and washed through western civilization, all begin and continue to depend upon flooding: the most ancient cultures of Europe and Asia were nurtured on the floodplains of the Nile, source of our most remote common ancestors from the heart of Africa, and from the Fertile Crescent of Mesopotamia, 'between the two rivers', Tigris and Euphrates. Prior to that, thousands of years even before the Axial Age, ancient peoples migrated from the Levant to the Black Sea, to the mouth of the Danube, which they named for a primordial goddess of Neolithic civilization 'Anu' – hence Danube – Anu's river of life, whose courses they followed throughout Europe, settling on her shores, westwards through the Balkans, Hungary, Austria, Germany; southwards along the Rhone to the Camargue and Marseilles; northwards along the Rhine, into Denmark – Danumark – the country named for her; further westwards to England, where Anu becomes Avon, and into Ireland where it becomes Abhainn, and eventually in a modern-ancient iteration of perpetual recurrence and beginning-again, as James Joyce's (1995) Anna Livia Plurabelle – the river of life, river of manifold beauties, which, 'by a commodious vicus of recirculation' may enable us all to begin again …

> All valid ideals are already anchored in a deep tradition, in ways of life which have already been lived. They cannot enter history like a newly invented plan that sweeps reality aside or shapes it from above. The validly new is a recreation of a tradition.
>
> Taylor 2007: 748

This is exactly Joyce's formulation, a formulation that he takes from Vico: 'imagination is nothing but the working over of what is remembered … imagination is memory' (Joyce, in Ellmann, 1983). This is how Joyce works with the traces of deep memory that find expression in everyday speech to cultivate imaginative resources for a new future. Joyce's vocation is to look and to listen for the transcendent ideal that is incarnated in the mundane immanent reality as it is encoded in deep traditions and expressed in the ordinary language of everyday life, and to bring it into the light to illuminate the coming – already present – dark age.

From pleonexic isolism to sympathetic resonance?

Throughout this volume we have analysed and diagnosed severe disorders that are haunting contemporary society. We have done so by providing a general framework of understanding, and then moved on to analysing three specific ills that affects human beings across the generational scale, from young people, through adults to seniors. Now, the theoretical perspectives used in those analyses are not the same but some of the theoretical undertones are. That is, the overall diagnosis rests on the presumption that we are dealing with a civilizational problem, thereby enabling us to direct our focus to social pathologies of contemporary civilization.

In this final chapter we have mentioned a wide variety of critical aspects of our contemporary civilization that seems to support the emergence of these social pathologies. One of them is pleonexia. In his fine book specifically on pleonexia, while discussing the images Socrates uses to understand and characterize the phenomenon in question, one of the contributors to this volume – Dany-Robert Dufour – writes the following.

> He [Socrates, ed.] compares those who indulge in feelings of always wanting more with the plover, this bird that eats and defecates at the same time. Because it can never get enough. Today, one could put it otherwise: The pleonexic – he, who always wants more (money, in this case) is an 'addict'. An addict who, like the drug-addict, always wants more because he is always in a state of craving. But what also becomes visible here, on the horizon, is the punishment: the destruction, or rather self-destruction of the intemperate.
>
> Dufour 2015: 22–3

Socrates' image, which Dufour presents here, is strong and resounding. If we keep on supporting the economical and socio-political strategies and policies that demand us to follow the rules of pleonexia, we are following a path towards self-destruction. Excess, and ever more excess, is the force creating addiction and hence leading us to self-destruction. Perhaps this image is pertinent to use when trying to encapsulate the overall state of contemporary civilization. Instead of finding secure grounds we are constantly undermining the stability of the foundation on which we should rest. But if this image is correct, it also leaves us with a duty to envisage something else than what we are facing today.

In order to be able to move towards this 'something else' and revolutionize our lives, or rather, in order to retune them, or let them be retuned, we need to take, says Dufour, 'conserving measures' (Dufour 2011: 305). What is needed, above all, is not so much a long march through the institutions but a series of long walks through history. 'So it is a voyage through the grand narratives on which western civilization based itself that we need to undertake' (ibid.: 31). Things took certain turns in this history and certain things got lost. For instance: when Mandeville published his famous *Fable of the Bees* in 1704, a direct heir of Glaucon from Plato's *Politheia* raised his voice. The English Enlightenment, says Dufour, resumed the debate precisely at the point where Plato had closed it two millennia earlier (ibid.: 98). Plato rejected *pleonexia*, Mandeville enthroned it, Adam Smith legitimized it and De Sade celebrated it. And, in the course of the former century, the Sadean spirit came slowly but steadily and, finally, mightily upon us. 'We live in an increasingly Sadean world,' Dufour states in *La Cité Perverse* (Dufour 2009: 11). The subjectivity into which the individual is subjectivized today is an 'isolist' or 'Sadean' one, it involves a subject whose passions are liberated in order to be colonized and mobilized by the 'Divine Market'. Recovery from this – a renovation of retunement – can only come via recollection of what has been lost, a loss not so much of realities, but of possibilities. The individual, says Dufour, still has to arrive, and it may arrive 'after liberalism', after we have overcome that slavery, after we have retuned ourselves, or have ourselves become retuned. The 'isolist' individual then may turn into a 'sympathetic' one. Pleonexia and dysrhythmia may turn into sympathy and resonance. But this will take a long march through history, or rather a whole series of long walks. And it will also take a multiplicity of perspectives on what could be termed, following Foucault, the 'ontology of the present'.

So, although we have limited ourselves in this chapter to discussing certain directions one could follow when tackling the overall issue of social pathologies of contemporary civilization, we do not wish to limit our research programme to these themes and perspectives. In fact, we rather envisage a multidimensional and multidisciplinary programme that sets out to confront the social pathologies of contemporary civilization from various sources of inspiration. Our overall idea – and hope – is thus that this book series will cover a variegated ground in the necessary pursuit to analyse and contextualize the malaises of contemporary civilization.

Notes

1 Goya's famous (1799) etching *El sueño de la razón produce monstruos* is mistranslated, for *sueño* does not mean 'sleep' of reason, but rather 'dream', as in the fantasy/wish; so it is 'the *dream* of reason produces monsters'.
2 For further discussion of pleonexia in the context of neoliberalism in Ireland, see Keohane and Kuhling 2014.
3 For further discussion of Orion as a figure of deregulation and the neoliberal revolution, see Keohane 2014.

4 Ghasemzadeh, N. and Maziar-Zafari, A. (2011): 'A brief journey into the history of the arterial pulse'. *Cardiology Research and Practice*, 2011(164832); http://www.hindawi.com/journals/crp/2011/164832 (accessed 14 June 2016).
5 Joseph Conrad's *Heart of Darkness* was inspired by his meeting Roger Casement, an Irishman who was British Consul in West Africa, commissioned to report on atrocities against native workers in the rubber industry of the Congo Free State (later the Belgian Congo; later the Democratic Republic of the Congo). The ironically named Congo Free State was entirely the private property of Leopold II, King of the Belgians.
6 The key opposition in the popular TV series *The Walking Dead*, one could say, is that of the absolute egocentrism of the 'walkers' versus the mutual sympathy of the 'survivors', a sympathy which again and again has to be defended and regained.
7 Bolts of rough cotton, surplus production, used (as well as pieces of brass wire) as payment 'advances' to natives, thereby putting them in debt.
8 In this context perhaps we can understand Frantz Fanon (2004) (and indeed many radicalized young people in the *banlieux* of Brussels and Paris today) when, experiencing this profound dissonance he declares: 'so let us leave behind this Europe, which is never done talking about Man, but murders him wherever it meets him!'
9 A contemporary exemplary practice of this method is by Maggie O'Neill (O'Neill and Hubbard 2010), who does this kind of empathetic understanding by walking with vulnerable groups, such as street sex-workers, homeless people, migrants seeking to find themselves in new cities and, recently, with refugees.

References

Antonovsky, A. (1979): *Health, Stress and Coping*. San Francisco: Jossey-Bass.

Arendt, H. (2006/1963): *Eichmann in Jerusalem: A Report on the Banality of Evil*. London: Penguin Classics.

Balot, R.K. (2001a): *Greed and Injustice in Classical Athens*. Princeton, NJ: Princeton University Press.

Balot, R.K. (2001b): Aristotle's critique of Phaleas: justice, inequality and pleonexia. *Hermes*, 129 (1): 32–44.

Benjamin, W. (1977): A Berlin chronicle. In: Benjamin, *One Way Street*. London: Verso.

Benjamin, W. (1992): Theses on the philosophy of history. In: Benjamin, *Illuminations*. London: Fontana.

Berardi, F. (2012): *The Uprising: On Poetry and Finance*. Los Angeles, CA: Semiotext(e).

Casement, R. (1904): *Report from His Majesty's Consul at Boma Respecting the Administration of the Independent State of the Congo* [aka 'The Casement Report']. London: HM Stationary Office.

Casement, R. (1997/1910): *Roger Casement's Diaries – 1910 – the Black and the White*. Roger Sawyer (ed.). London: Pimlico.

Conrad, J. (2009/1899): *Heart of Darkness*. London: Oneworld Classics.

Dufour, D.-R. (2007): *Le Divin Marché. La Révolution Culturelle Libérale*. Paris: Éditions Denoël.

Dufour, D.-R. (2008): *The Art of Shrinking Heads: On the New Servitude of the Liberated in the Age of Total Capitalism*. Cambridge: Polity.

Dufour, D.-R. (2009): *La Cité Perverse. Libéralisme et Pornographie*. Paris: Éditions Denoël.

Dufour, D.-R. (2011): *L'Individu Qui Vient … Après le Libéralisme*. Paris: Éditions Denoël.

Dufour, D.-R. (2015): *Pléonexie*. Lormont: Le Bord de L'eau.

Ellmann, R. (1983): *James Joyce*. Oxford: Oxford University Press.

Eliot, T.S. (1991): The Hollow Men. In: *Collected Poems 1909–1962.* Orlando: Harcourt Brace.
Fanon, F. (2004): *The Wretched of the Earth.* New York: Grove Press.
Geertz, C. (1973): *The Interpretation of Cultures.* New York: Basic Books.
Gilloch, G. (1997): *Myth and Metropolis: Walter Benjamin and the City.* Cambridge: Polity Press.
Gramsci, A. (1971): *Selections from the Prison Notebooks.* London: Lawrence & Wishart.
Graves, R. (1960): *The Greek Myths vols. 1 and 2.* London: Penguin.
Hallam, L.A. (2012): *Screening the Marquis De Sade: Pleasure, Pain and the Transgressive Body in Film.* Jefferson, NC: McFarland & Co.
Haraway, D. (1989): A Manifesto for Cyborgs. In: Nicholson, L.J. (ed.), *Feminism/Postmodernism.* London: Routledge.
Heidegger. M. (1971): *Poetry, Language, Thought.* New York: Harper & Row.
Hochschild, A. (2012): *King Leopold's Ghost: A Story of Greed, Terror and Heroism in Colonial Africa.* London: Pan.
Hyde, L. (1998): *Trickster Makes this World: Mischief, Myth and Art.* New York: Farrar, Straus & Giroux.
James, W. (1890): *The Principles of Psychology.* New York: Holt.
Joyce, J. 199/1939): *Finnegans Wake.* London: Picador.
Jung, Carl, (1960): *The Structure and Dynamics of the Psyche.* Princeton, NJ: Princeton University Press.
Kant, I. (2002/1875): *Critique of Judgment.* Oxford; Oxford University Press.
Keohane, K. (2014): Possessing Utopia: a genealogical demonology. *Irish Journal of Anthropology*, 17(1): 18–26.
Keohane, K. and C. Kuhling (2014): Pleonexic tyranny in Plato's *Republic* and in the Irish Republic. In: Keohane and Kuhling, *The Domestic, Political and Moral Economies of Post Celtic Tiger Ireland: What Rough Beast?* Manchester: Manchester University Press.
Kerenyi, C. (1980): *The Gods of the Greeks.* London: Thames & Hudson.
Lacan, J. (1977): *Écrits: A Selection.* New York: W.W. Norton.
Lacan, J. (1991): *Speech and Language in Psychoanalysis*, translated, with notes and commentary by A. Wilden. Baltimore, MD: Johns Hopkins University Press.
Laclau, E. and C. Mouffe (1985): *Hegemony and Socialist Strategy.* London: Verso.
Mouffe, C. (1988): Radical democracy: modern or postmodern?. In: Ross, A. (ed.), *Universal Abandon? The Politics of Postmodernism.* Minneapolis: University of Minnesota Press.
Myers, K. (2011): Metanoia and the transformation of opportunity. *Rhetoric Studies Quarterly*, 41(1): 1–18.
Nietzsche, F. (1882/1873): On truth and lies in an extra moral sense. In: Kaufman, W. (ed.), *The Portable Nietzsche.* London: Penguin.
O'Neill, M. and Hubbard, P. (2010): Walking, sensing, belonging: ethno-mimesis as performative praxis. *Visual Studies*, 25(1): 46–58.
Plato (1997): *Republic*, translated by J.L. Davies and D.J. Vaughan. London: Wordsworth Editions.
Ransom, J.C. (1939): Yeats and his symbols. *Kenyon Review*, 1(3): 309–22.
Ricoeur, P. (1993): *The Rule of Metaphor.* Toronto: University of Toronto Press.
Salecl, R. (2011): *The Tyranny of Choice.* London: Profile.
Stiglitz, J. (2015): *An Interview with Nobel Laureate Joseph Stiglitz: The Loss of the American Dream, Trickle Down Economics and Free Trade*, presented by General Economic

Dynamics, 6 October 2015. In: https://ged-project.de/topics/competitiveness/an-interview-with-nobel-laureate-joseph-stiglitz (accessed 25 June 2016).
Taylor, C. (1991): The skilled pastor. *Augsburg Fortress*, 8: 64.
Taylor, C. (2007): *A Secular Age*. Cambridge, MA: Harvard University Press.
Thomassen, B. (2013) Modernity as spiritual disorder: searching for a vocabulary of social pathologies in the work of Erik Voegelin. In: Keohane, K. and Petersen, A. (eds), *The Social Pathologies of Contemporary Civilization*. London: Ashgate: 43–59.
Trench, R. (2006/1880): *Synonyms of the New Testament*. London: Macmillan, 9th edition, 255-261.
Vico, G. (1999/1744): *New Science*. London: Penguin.
Wittgenstein, L. (1994/1958): *Philosophical Investigations*. London: Blackwell.
Wright Mills, C. (1959): *The Sociological Imagination*. Oxford: Oxford University Press.

Index